MW01487198

www.BramcostPublications.com

ISBN 10: 1-934268-83-6
ISBN 13: 978-1-934268-83-4

Library of Congress Control Number: 2008937886

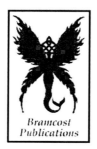

Bramcost
Publications

Creative Hair Styling

by

Alfred Morris

Professor British Hairdressers' Academy

International Hairdressers' Society

La Société du Progrès de la Coiffure

Hon. Professor Institute de Belgique

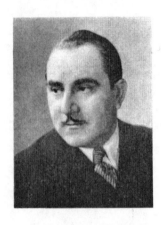

Mr. ALFRED MORRIS

Principal of the

MORRIS SCHOOL OF HAIRDRESSING and BEAUTY CULTURE LTD.

and

LONDON INSTITUTE OF HAIRDRESSING and BEAUTY CULTURE

6 SHAFTESBURY AVENUE
PICCADILLY CIRCUS
LONDON, W.1

Author of " Successful Water Waving "

President:
The International Hairdressers' Society
(London) 1930-1934

Highest Awards in Open Competitions

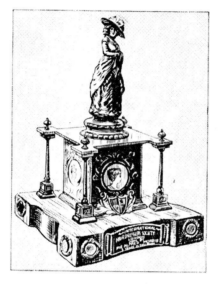

The American
Championship
Gold Cup
won outright
Chicago 1938

The International
200 gns. Challenge Trophy
won 3 years in succession
1928—1929—1930

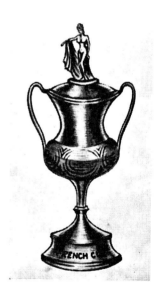

French Challenge
Cup won
1929

Grand Prix. Hair Styling (Hairdressers' Exhibition)
and Holder of 40 Gold Medals and Diplomas

3

Acknowledgements

The purpose of this book is to encourage and assist readers to gain experience and confidence, and to increase your knowledge, so that each and every one of you will be a credit to the hairdressing profession.

I wish to express my thanks to all those who have helped me to present this publication in a concise and instructive manner, but particularly to Miss Esme Limburg, a tutor at the Morris School, for her drawings and illustrations, my teaching staff, and the following well-known hair designers for kindly vetting my script to ensure that the technical information is authentic, practical and helpful.

Mr. Joseph Pou, acclaimed European Champion by winning the Fellowship Gold Star, Lyceum, London, 1947.

Mr. Julius Liverani, winner Grand Prix Hair Styling Contest, Paris, 1946.

Alfred George Scott, Chief Hair Stylist, British National Film Studios, Elstree. Twice winner of £500 gold trophy and winner of Grand Prix Hair Styling Contest, Olympia, 1938.

Alfred Morris

TABLE OF CONTENTS

7

Introduction

O^N placing before the hairdressing trade my second book, I have been able to publish much instructive material which has long been buried among the purely technical information with which it was surrounded.

I have not tried to write extravagantly, but have endeavoured to express my ideals as simply as possible. I trust that the attention I have given to the subject and my long experience of teaching have enabled me to pass on useful information to others ; and confidently believe that this book will help to improve their knowledge of the wonderful art of creative hairdressing.

This art has existed for ages. Sometimes it is left to individual taste, which in some cases may be right, in others wrong. But to make hairdressing an art it must be based on artistic principles which in turn are based on fundamentals so far as technicalities are concerned. To assist in this, carefully-prepared illustrations will define the leading principles of technique which will form the basis in preparing perfectly-balanced designs. Every sketch is authentic and simply explained, so that a student or an experienced hairdresser will be able to follow each movement.

I sincerely hope that everyone who studies the information given, will be patient and persistent, for this publication endeavours to meet the need for technical guidance. I believe this book will inspire confidence and help you to achieve your ambition to become an artistic hairdresser. Finally, should you not achieve perfect results immediately—persevere. Success will follow, and to quote the words of Ruskin:—" It is the effort that deserves praise, not the success, nor is it a question whether students are more clever or more dull than others, but whether they have done the best with the gifts they have."

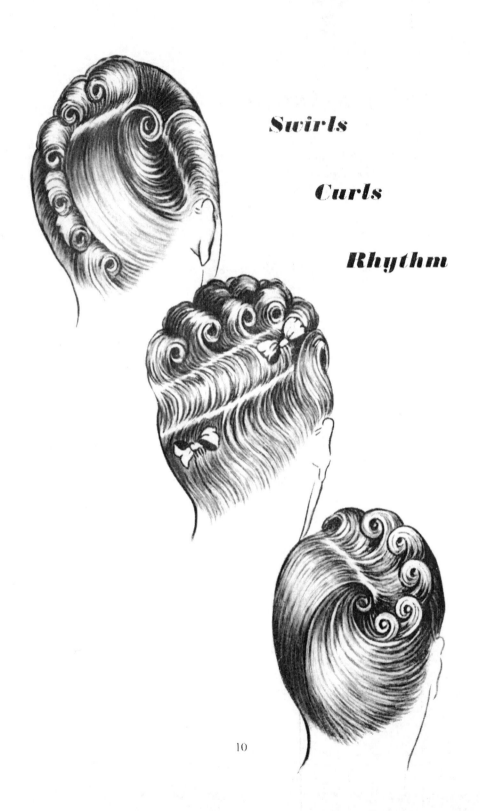

Swirls

Curls

Rhythm

10

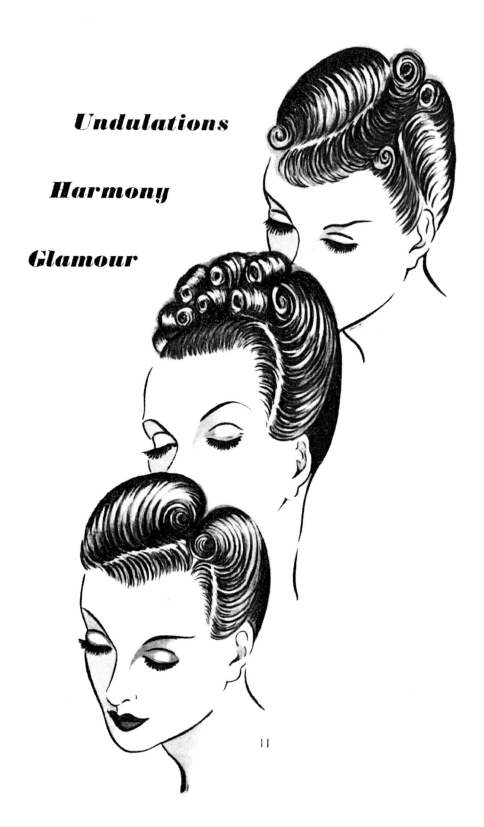

Undulations

Harmony

Glamour

11

CHAPTER ONE

General Principles

HAIRDRESSING styles have developed over a long period, and to-day we have designs of soft, artistic beauty. With such a variety of hairdressing styles the modern woman is not considered well-dressed unless her hair is also well groomed.

Every woman endeavours to look her best. It is for you to show the client that you understand her requirements; you must always study individuality. A suitable style cannot be achieved unless you look into the mirror and observe your client's features. Comb the lady's hair into different positions--right off her ears, showing half the ears, well forward on the face, well forward over the forehead; comb the hair up at the back and observe the shape of the neckline, and so on.

Your client will be impressed immediately by this proof that you are not only an experienced hairdresser, but also an artist who is deciding on the most suitable style for her.

No matter how artistic a hairdresser may be, the client usually terminates the session with her own suggestions on the way her hair should be dressed. The hairdresser cannot dictate on a question of style; it is a matter for the client, but the hairdresser should be prepared to carry out any style to give satisfaction. This is why the fundamental principles of various methods of styling are important. You will find that a number of your clients do not respond to the introduction of a new hair style merely because it may not seem to them to be practical. Almost invariably you will hear them say:—" I could never wear that style."

In other words, after the hairdresser has finished the dressing, the client may be unable to re-dress that particular style herself. Many of my readers will admit this to be correct, but there is a tremendous difference between a practical dressing and an elaborate style. A pretty and artistic style can be practical; as an example see Fig. 140. This dressing could easily be called a practical one. The wearer could manipulate her hair and recomb it into position.

You will often have to design a style suitable for the client's new hat. The style must obviously be your own version, but one suitable to the wearer as well as adaptable to the hat.

Milliners have themselves been the creators of hair fashion, and we have had to fall into line with them. The hats in vogue for the last few years, for example, have shown only one side of the head, or have been placed on the crown, exposing the entire front line. It is vital to the wearers of these hats that the hair is dressed accordingly.

GENERAL PRINCIPLES

Hairdressing is one of the chief factors in the designs of to-day. The milliners study the latest coiffures and make their designs to harmonise with them.

The many fashions of the modern milliners' art, with their revealing lines and subtle simplicity, demand that we hairdressers give the finishing touch to the *tout ensemble*. It is we who finally and triumphantly reveal the elegance of the milliners' art.

All hairdressers strive to become artists. Sometimes their work is jeopardised because their clientele are not accustomed to styles other than those that are merely practical. Even in a working-class district, where clients demand solid waves and curls that must remain in for some time, there are always a few who want artistry as well. From experience I have found that students who have been used to this type of clientele can easily adapt themselves to the finer arts of styling.

The chapter on basic principles will show you how to incorporate my knowledge in this most artistic branch of our craft. I hope that readers will not only interest themselves when they practise these designs, but will also introduce them to their clients. The introduction of something new is always good propaganda, especially among clients who talk about their hair. Enormous possibilities are at your disposal if you are capable of justifying the demands of these coiffures. Fresh activity, repeated activity, are the secrets of success.

Many articles on hairdressing are published in the press. Fashion committees try to incorporate designs that are practical and artistic. We know, of course, that this is what we all desire, but hairdressing cannot be a definite or standardized style, since coiffures will always be given individuality by one's own interpretation. Information derived from newspapers tends to make women more hair conscious.

> **"Create Fashions,**
> **Evolve Fashions,**
> **Follow Fashions,**
> ***Wisdom."***

> **"Stray From Fashion,**
> ***Folly."***

CHAPTER TWO

Shampooing and the Preparing of the Hair

IT is impossible to carry out an attractive design unless the hair is in a really clean and healthy condition. The ever-increasing demand upon the hairdresser for artistic styles gives us infinite scope, but success lies in the preparation of the hair before styling.

Cleanliness makes hair pliable for setting; the dressing-out is made easier, and back-combing can be more successfully achieved. Nowadays, there should be no excuse for unruly or dull hair after shampooing. Scientific products such as reconditioning shampoo creams, water soluble oils, and soapless shampoos enhance beautiful coiffures. These modern hair-cleansing preparations form soluble compounds with the calcium and magnesium salts in hard water, and are thus ideal for washing bleached or dyed hair, since no scum is formed to cling to the hair shafts, and to leave the hair dull and sticky. Consequently, after washing *any* head with such cleansing preparations, there is no necessity for a final acetic acid rinse.

During a shampoo with some soap shampoos the hair shaft may become coated with soap scum. Ordinary water, unless it is softened by an effective plant, contains a proportion of calcium and magnesium salts. These form insoluble compounds with soap and adhere to bleached hair because of the somewhat roughened condition of the hair shaft. This causes the hair to tangle, robs it of its lustre and makes a clean setting impossible. Being insoluble in water, the scum cannot be washed away no matter how much rinsing the hair receives; and it is only after further preparation that the operator can bring the hair into a suitable condition for setting.

One way of overcoming this difficulty is to add about two teaspoonsful of ordinary acetic acid to a quart of warm water, and use this solution as a final rinse after the shampoo. Another method is to use one of the proprietary after-shampoo rinses, but the progressive hairdresser uses a good soapless shampoo, especially in districts where the water is hard. This eliminates all these problems.

Setting hair that has been bleached or dyed always presents some difficulty because the hair when wet tends to cling together and the operator finds it difficult to comb. To minimise the tendency of the hair to cling to the comb, a few drops of brilliantine, or a small quantity of reconditioning cream rubbed between the palms of the hands and then over the hair, will distribute a very fine oily film over each and every hair. This will ensure easy combing. Nevertheless, it is strongly recommended that the hair be combed out from the ends first; this prevents pulling, and there is less chance of breaking the hair.

Bleached hair must be treated differently from ordinary hair. When hair has been bleached the hair shafts will cling together; the hair is more porous and will absorb a greater quantity of water. This accounts for the increased time such hair takes to dry. It is, therefore, an advantage to remove all excess water with a towel after washing, and a spirit lotion applied to the hair for setting will hasten the drying period.

In conclusion, I must stress two very important points about bleached hair:—

1. *Never have the water too hot when shampooing.*
2. *Never allow your client to remain too long in a very hot hood drier.*

CHAPTER THREE

Shaping and Tapering for Successful Styling

CREATIONS of styles that are practical, becoming and fashionable, serve as a foundation for success in hairdressing. Simple but well-carried-out designs offer an ideal opportunity to combine the three things most desired by clients—practicality, becomingness and fashion.

Careful observance of a few fundamental principles of preparing the hair prior to styling, is of paramount importance. Before a coiffure can be designed, the hair must of course be properly thinned and tapered. Variation and graduation of different lengths of hair for a particular style are the secrets of successful styling. Clients must be educated to this way of thinking, and the hairdresser must explain that when the hair is properly tapered it is more pliable and the set lasts much longer. Cleverly-cut hair almost moulds into a style; as a result, the hair can be set twice as fast as usual and the combing-out is comparatively much more simple. Drying time is also saved because the excess bulk of hair has been removed. In cutting and tapering for a particular style, it is very important to keep in mind throughout the entire process the finished head-dress.

There is a variety of hair styles for the hairdresser to choose from; short hair moulded closely to the contours of the head; " Bangs " softly waved or curled; an array of " puff " curls on the top; a one-sided " Edwardian "; a sleek " Page Boy " or hair simply-waved back with loose fluffy curls. But shaping and shortening the hair are the first steps. This may not necessarily mean a great reduction in length, since you may want the hair adaptable for a number of styles, but it will mean considerable reduction in bulk.

Hair-shaping is an art that requires study and expert tuition. One can speak of the art of haircutting only when such essential points as the style and shape have been chosen. There are a considerable number of hairdressers who care very little, or not at all, about the preparation of the hair; but if the hairdresser is not interested in his work, he has surely missed his vocation, since the craft of hairdressing must be inspired by genuine interest. It is the hairdresser's job to discover the style which suits his client best, and he should learn how the hair should be cut and tapered accordingly. To accomplish this, the hairdresser will first have to consider the general appearance—the shape of the head, the fullness of the hair, and its quality and texture. It is the thickness, however, which is most important. It is this which determines the cut, but the texture plays only a conditional role, as thick but soft hair is comparatively easy to manage, while thick and coarse hair is far more difficult.

Women appreciate a good smart head-dress, and the hairdresser must introduce the necessary modifications. The first of these modifications consists of giving the head the right shape, which is best achieved by tapering. Cutting the hair to the desired length is the first procedure. Once this is completed, then the tapering can be done.

Tapering can be carried out with an ordinary pair of scissors, a razor or tapering scissors.

If the scissors are allowed to slither along separate sections, the hair is cut to different

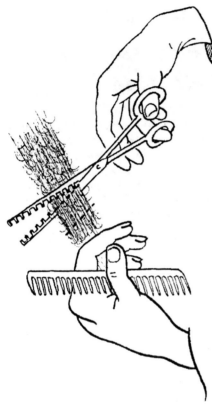

Fig. I.
Hair back-combed, dotted lines indicating
first incision.

lengths, so that the strands are tapered and the desired length is achieved.

The razor taper requires more skill and practise; with the razor, the hair can be tapered down almost to the roots. This forms an excellent foundation for the top hair to rest upon, which is essential if it is desired to give a *lift* to the dressing.

A further advantage of the razor taper is that it allows the tackling of any hair length. Razor cutting should be done while the hair is damp, and should be tapered underneath the hair if the hair is being combed down, or on the top if the hair is combed up. Always hold the mesh between the second and third fingers while cutting. Begin at the roots, bringing the razor towards you. As the razor must be manipulated from the wrist, pressure with the razor must not be too heavy.

It is sometimes said that the advantage of the razor technique is preferable for thick, especially curly hair, but this is not so, for scientifically-done razor hair-cutting will certainly enhance the charm of good hair-dressing.

A scientific taper can be achieved by mechanical means. The introduction of tapering scissors has been a great boon to the hairdresser. If properly used, this method is, in my opinion, the best way of tapering, but certain principles must be followed. Although the incision should be invisible, there must be plenty of hair to be combed out.

It is advisable, however, to follow certain fundamentals which are explained in the accompanying sketch (Fig. 1). From the very first cut, the practical advantage is obvious; but the main point, which applies in any method of tapering, is always to bear in mind the desired shape, since this is the chief object of a taper. Short hair has made tapering particularly popular; with the present-day modes a scientific hair taper is compatible with the modern ideas of hair beauty and hair culture, and it seems to express the present-day tendency towards realism. Would it not be better to adapt this strong realism to the achieving of natural perfection and beauty by trying to create the impression of fullness of hair where it does not exist? Tapering will create fullness because of its pliability, and the thinness of the hair is successfully concealed.

The tapering scissors are held with the thumb and third finger of the right hand. The action of slowly opening and closing the blades of the scissors offers about double the resistance of ordinary scissors, accompanied by a distinct feeling of each tooth engaging

16

with a corresponding tooth of the other blade. Should the hair be very thick, and require drastic tapering, the full complement of teeth along the lengths of the scissor blades will have to interlock.

During my experience of teaching, certain principles have been modified, particularly the method of tapering. When one is taught a certain method it is usual to continue that method until another device is introduced.

When tapering scissors were first introduced, everyone began the first incision at the roots. I adopted this method and taught students accordingly, but now my principle of tapering with tapering scissors—one which I consider to be far more scientific and practical—is to begin at the points instead of at the roots. The top hair should not be tapered so much as the underneath hair. For instance, should a large swirled movement be wanted, either at the front or at the sides, the top layer should be divided off and left until last, for no matter how careful you may be when tapering, a certain amount of short hair may show.

Back-combing, prior to tapering, is of great importance, because it enables the hair to be tapered in entirely different lengths. As an example, take a strand of hair and make a direct incision with the tapering scissors, then comb it, and you will see that where the incision has been made, short stumps of hair will show through. Now take another strand, back-comb it, make an incision, and you will then observe that no short hair is seen. The accompanying sketch shows the scissors being inserted on a slant. A number of readers will disagree with the idea of beginning the tapering at the points, but when they study the reason they will no doubt agree that the principle is far more scientific. When the hair is cut at the roots first, the hair combed out and another incision made higher up, then the principle is correct, but the majority of hairdressers begin tapering at the roots and gradually work towards the points. In my opinion, the hair cannot be properly tapered this way because every incision, except the first one, is futile, as the already tapered hair is tapered over and over again. My method is totally different. By beginning at the points and working up to the roots a carefully-balanced scientific taper is produced.

CHAPTER FOUR

The Art of Curling

THROUGH the ages the majority of women have always curled their hair. A coiffure which incorporates curls placed in different positions always has a softening effect upon the features and creates a more youthful appearance.

Years ago women curled their hair with papers or rags; even to-day many women use "curlers" without realizing the damage they do to the hair. It is very difficult to obtain a curl which continues to the point of the hair in this way; almost invariably the ends are merely bent sharply in one direction or another, eventually becoming very brittle, causing the hair to split or break and generally retarding its growth.

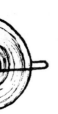

Fig. 2

By keeping a strand of hair as flat to the head as possible and holding it taut with one hand while curling it from the point upwards with the other, the perfect pin curl may be achieved. The pin curl is round and smooth, with no twists in it, and its circumference fits its own square base at the scalp, upon which it is pinned. The tips of the strand of hair form a very tight centre to create the apex of the curl.

A frequent fault is that of spoiling the shape of a well-formed curl by placing the pins in carelessly and thereby marking it. Two pins should be inserted gently from right to left, as illustrated (Fig. 2), without pushing them right in, as the head of the pin would then cause an indenture to the curl. This procedure would be reversed with a left-handed operator.

When pinning-up rows of curls, the pins should be kept parallel with the rows. The prongs of the pins will then be found to extend into the adjacent curls, thereby helping the whole row to stay in position. Unless the rows of curls are made from left to right, the pins will project into hair which still has to be curled up.

For some styles curls that stand away from the head are necessary. These are made in a similar way to the ordinary pin curl, but, instead of being placed flat to the head, are pinned at right-angles to it, going in an upward direction, or conversely, downwards.

Hold the curl with the left hand, take a pin with the right hand, and, while holding the head of it with the first finger and thumb, open the prongs of the pin with the middle finger. One prong is placed one side of the curl, and one the other side, the ends of the prongs reaching to the centre of the curl, where they are pinched together between the thumb and the first finger of the left hand, while being thrust through the remainder of the curl with the right hand. Another pin is placed similarly, in the opposite direction to the previous one, thereby forcing both pins to interlock and keep the curl in position (Fig. 3).

For similar curls turned *upwards*, a third pin is used to hold the curl to the head, otherwise the curl would fall away when the fingers were removed. The placing of a net over curls of this type must be done carefully to prevent them turning side-ways and thus spoiling the desired result.

18

Ordinary pin curls can be made in two directions only, clockwise and counter-clockwise; and, for clarity throughout this book, the abbreviation "*C*" for clockwise, and "*CC*" for counterclockwise will be used. For clarity, too, the part of the hair of a pincurl which is growing from the roots of the head will be termed the *Stem* of the curl. The direction given to a strand of hair before it is curled, determines the *position* of the *Stem*. By making *C* or *CC* curls, so that their stems are in varied positions, different styles may be obtained.

On page 20 is a simple chart to which the student should refer when attempting to place curls in their correct positions for various styles.

A *SWIRL* curl is given a long curved stem, at the top of which is pinned a *C* or *CC* curl. To form a good curve to the stem, and to ensure flatness to the head, an irregular base is made at the scalp by taking the partings on an upward slant, always making sure that the front of the base is longer than the back part of it. See Figs. 5 and 6. In a movement requiring two or more swirl curls for

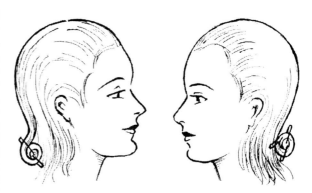

Fig. 3.   Showing curls pinned at right-angles to the head, going in an upward and downward direction.

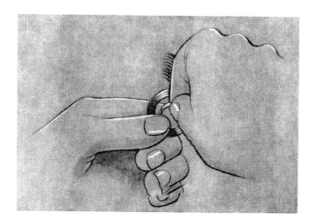

Fig. 4.   The process of making a *CC* curl

its formation, all the curls must overlap the stems and partings of the previous swirl curls to prevent breaks from showing in the finished dressing.

At present, the method of obtaining waves by the dressing out of pin-curls is widely used and is certainly a useful practice when a full movement is desired; waves obtained in this manner do not lie as flat to the head as those placed "*en pli*"* with the fingers and comb. This method of waving is termed *Reverse Curling*.

Let me repeat that there are only two types of pin curls, *C* or *CC*. There is in fact no such thing as a reverse curl! It is an ordinary *C* or *CC* curl when put "*en pli*." When it is dressed out, however, it is turned first one way and then the other, thereby continually *reversing* the direction of the curl and obtaining waves from it.

If a curl is pinned to the head, dried slightly, the pins then removed and the curl allowed

* "*En pli*."   The preparation of setting waves and curls.

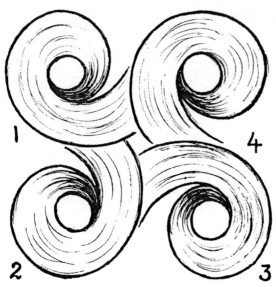

Fig. 5.   C Curls showing direction of Stems

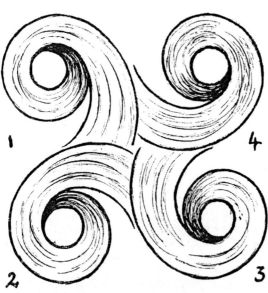

Fig. 6.   CC Curls showing direction of Stems

to drop out, as it drops it turns to one side and then the other, forming undulations. The waves would be larger near the roots than those towards the end of the strand of the hair, because the centre of the pin-curl has a smaller circumference than the outer part. Consequently waves uneven in size tend to result. To prevent this happening, pin-curls which are intended to be reverse curls when dressed out must be made with very large centres to them so that the resulting waves will be as even in size as possible. See Fig. 7.

If rows of curls all going in the same direction are pinned up in this fashion, and care is taken to make each curl comparatively even in size with the others, very natural and well-formed waves will be the result.

If, however, the same effect is required but with deeper undulations, the rows of curls may be pinned in alternate directions. The first row of curls being C, and the second row CC, as in Fig. 7, or vice-versa. In this way, *the stems* of the curls will be going straight from the scalp into the direction of the waves, causing the waves to be deeper than if all the curls were going in one direction. The crest of the waves will always fall in between the rows of curls, since a wave is, figuratively speaking, half of a circle or curl. Where large waves are needed with deep crests to them, one row of curls is made in one direction, while the next *two* rows are pinned with the curls going the opposite way. The crests of the waves will then fall in between the rows of curls which are going alternate ways, the two rows which go in one direction forming a large wave.

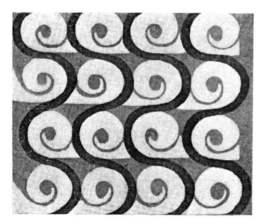

Fig. 7. Alternate rows of Curls, first row being clockwise

When dressing out from the Reverse Curl method, the hair is dried, brushed and combed right out. The waves are then placed in with the fingers and comb, as if finger-waving wet hair. The main points to remember about the art of curling are the following:—Curls must be made smoothly, with clean partings for their bases, and practical commonsense applied when carrying out different hair styles. Where a large movement is desired, *large* curls will be made for that particular movement; similarly, small curls will be made to create a tight effect; and when the Reverse Curl method is applied, the centres of the curls must be made as open as possible to ensure evenness of size in the resulting waves. Fig. 8 shows another method of curling, but on this occasion it is done with bigoudis; the curls are known as croquignole. These bigoudis are made with fairly thick paper cut in strips about 2½-3 inches wide and rolled up, the ends being fastened down with adhesive so that they will not unroll. Wherever the curls are required, take a piece of hair evenly divided off, and roll up to the head, placing pins as shown. Great care should be taken to make certain that the points are rolled on the curler in the first instance. When dressing these curls out, back-comb from the root to point, and with the aid of a postiche brush, brush up smoothly and roll over with a tail comb, with the

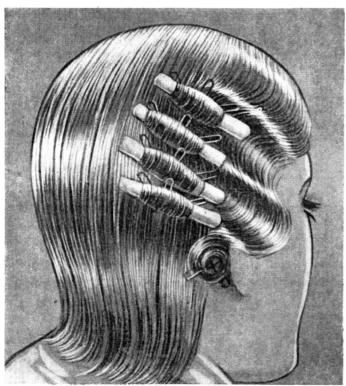

Fig. 8.

21

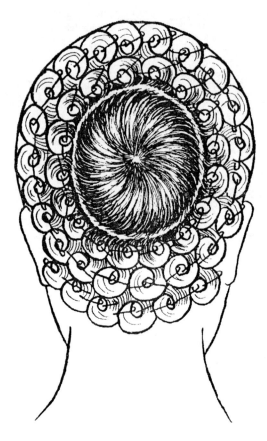

Fig. 9. Showing hair combed away from a central focus, and placed into a circular crest. CC Curls are placed up to the crest, whilst the other rows of Curls are Clockwise.

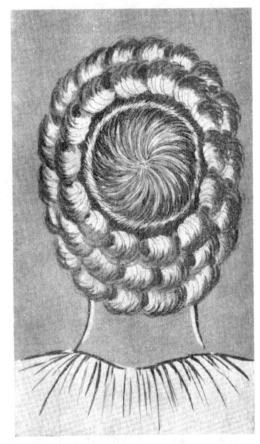

first finger. Before releasing finger, comb the hair over it, this will make the curl more secure owing to the hair having had back-combing; release finger and spread to whatever size required.

Fig. 10. Back dressing completed, with Puff Curls arranged round the Crest.

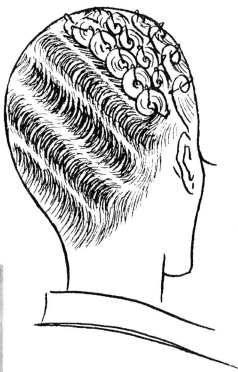

Fig. 11. Hair swathed from left to right in diagonal waves going upwards, ending in two rows of CC Curls.

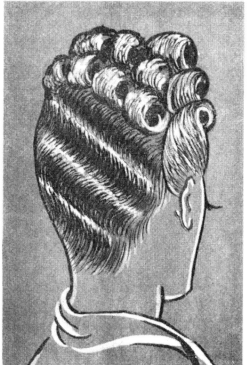

Fig. 12. Back dressing completed, with waves smoothed into position, and Puff Curls on the crown of the head.

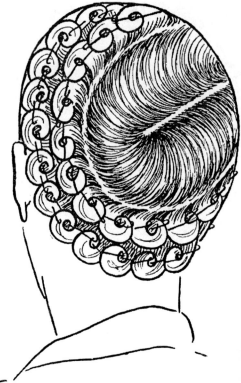

Fig. 13. Hair combed away from slanting parting on both sides, and swept into a semi-circular crest. *CC* Curls pinned up to this crest, with a second row of *C* Curls placed in position.

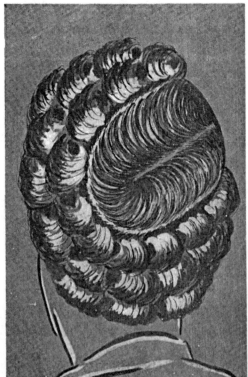

Fig. 14. Completed back dressing, with curls puffed out and arranged around the crest.

Fig. 15. Hair swept towards the face at sides, and straight down at the back, with two rows of curls also going towards face, at the sides. Tape placed in position to create shape at nape of neck, and two rows of curls at right angles to head pinned into position, the first row being pinned over the tape.

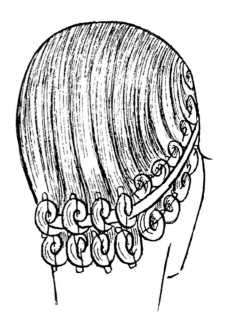

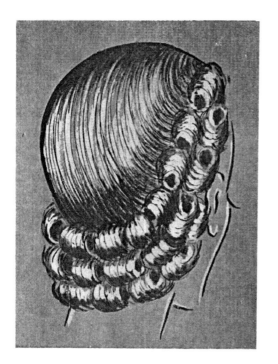

Fig. 16. Hair dressed out at back and sides, showing deep indenture at nape of neck, and back curls standing away from the head.

CHAPTER FIVE

The Art and Practice of Water-Waving

THE hairdresser is more in demand to-day than ever. That demand is mostly for water waving, and the public have been so educated that they know, when a hairdresser begins to set, whether the result will be good, bad or merely indifferent.

Because the public are so educated, the hairdresser must make a closer study of the subject. In water-waving there is wide scope for individuality, and if you work efficiently you need never fear your competitor. Water-waving is the first thing to learn before one becomes a stylist. I know a number of hairdressers who can style and shape hair expertly but who find it more difficult to place the hair in a commercial set.

Before we discuss hair-styling I shall explain the technique of setting hair and shall incorporate sketches and material taken from my previous publication, *Successful Water-Waving*. The basic principles are for the beginner. They are based on rules which are taught in the Morris School and which are easily translated and adapted.

To explain the origin of water-waving we must go back a number of years. It antedates Marcel Waving by a considerable period, and its use is not confined to living hair. It was originally practised for dressing postiche. The ultimate result of a water-wave depends on its lasting quality as well as on its beauty.

There are three types of hair—the naturally wavy hair, the permanently-waved hair and the straight hair.

Naturally wavy hair, which is the hairdresser's delight to set, will respond to any treatment in setting if it is not the negroid type, which comes under the category of frizzy hair. A good permanently-waved head can be water-waved almost as easily as naturally wavy hair. With naturally wavy hair, or good permanently-waved hair, it is possible to comb the hair back in a wet state, push the hair forward and obtain waves. This is called fashioning a wave. A water-wave is a thing of beauty, but if certain fundamentals are forgotten it will only remain beautiful so long as it is not combed. It must have a foundation of basic principles.

There are times when it is necessary to water-wave a frizzy or kinky perm. With this type of hair it is impossible to fashion a wave. The hair has to be prepared before setting. To do this a thick setting lotion or a little vaseline or petroleum jelly must be applied, and the hair brushed flat. The setting must be done very flat, the hair combed well, and the hairdresser must be certain that the hair is combed through to the scalp.

Straight hair always creates difficulties in water-waving. It is impossible to make the wave remain in very long. Straight hair must be thoroughly tapered to make the hair more pliable. In another chapter, water-waving with setting combs is explained, and this method is recommended for straight hair.

To acquire the technique of water-waving it is advisable to begin at the beginning. The following equipment is necessary for the learner: a Marteaux, preferably wavy, about 3 inches wide and approximately 12 inches long—tapered; a malleable block; an iron or wooden stand as shown in Fig. 17. Pin the Marteaux on to the block, wet the hair thoroughly and comb flat. If the hair is a little frizzy add about a teaspoonful of acetic acid to about a pint of hot water and apply to the hair. A little brilliantine before water-waving is also very helpful for fluffy hair. Place the block at an angle of, say, 45 degrees, as in Fig. 18, then comb the hair to the right or left in a semi-circular position, making sure that the comb is kept in a straight position all the time. The teeth of the comb should touch the block gently, at right angles to it when shaping a wave; but as soon as the forefinger is holding the crest in position, the comb must be turned completely sideways to comb the mesh right to the ends (see Fig. 19). This process stretches the hair between the teeth and bar of the comb, thus ensuring smoothness in the resulting waves.

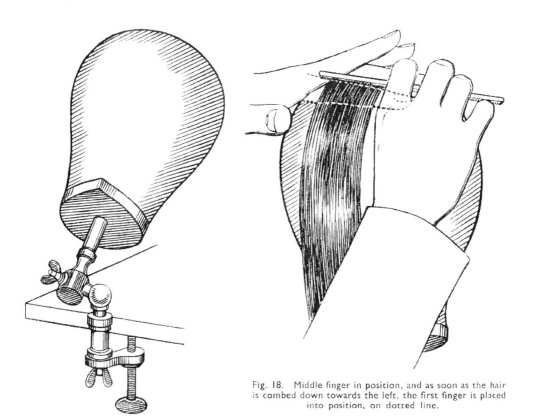

Fig. 17.

Fig. 18. Middle finger in position, and as soon as the hair is combed down towards the left, the first finger is placed into position, on dotted line.

27

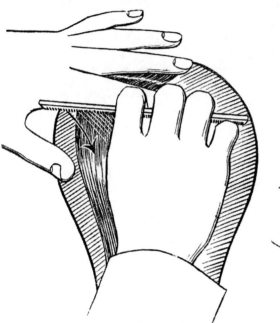

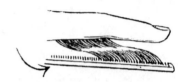

Fig. 20. Comb must always be kept parallel with finger.

Fig. 19. Arrow shows position of combed hair, as soon as the first finger is in position.

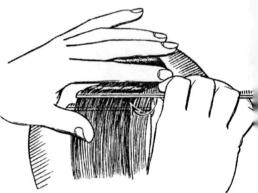

Fig. 22. Hair combed from the finger in a semi-circular movement indicated by arrow.

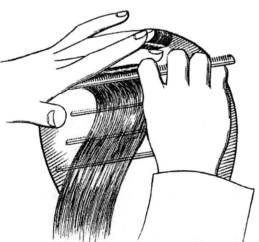

Fig. 21. Showing position of middle finger, with comb placed directly underneath, then moved towards the right. Replace first finger. Hair is then combed towards the left.

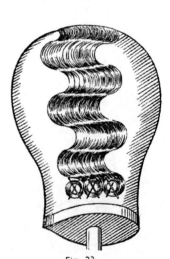

Fig. 23. Completed Marteaux.

CHAPTER SIX

The Hair Line and Practical Setting

The Technique of Water-Waving

HAIRDRESSING styles have developed over a long period, and to-day we have designs of soft and artistic beauty. I am not suggesting that the styles of years ago were very heavy—on the contrary—but the importance of scientific manipulation of the technicalities relating to water-waving is of the utmost importance and must be taught before styling is approached.

This gives me considerable scope, as it deals with the preliminary to my Step-by-Step method of technical water-waving as taught to the students of the Morris School of Hair-dressing.

Fig. 24 illustrates the hair combed right back, thus showing in detail the front hair line. You will observe that the hair grows lowest opposite the nose in the centre of the front hair line, then recedes over the eye, grows forward on the temples and again recedes below the temples in the same shape as the eye—in fact, parallel with the eye—and then the finish of the hair line is a V shape just below the eye level in front of the ear.

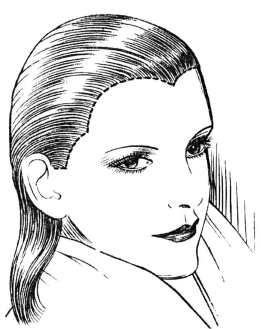

Fig. 24. Hair line showing peak and receding part over eyes—hair on temples and receding again level with eye—the end of hair line forming V shape.

Practical Setting

We are dealing with a left side parting, and the waves require setting parallel with the parting, and the design required is the three wave mode, as in Fig. 30. Comb the hair back on both sides, apply a little setting lotion (the latter makes the hair more pliable and hastens the drying as it contains spirit). The first movement is the backward wave, which means that the hair is combed with an upward movement as in Fig. 25. Place the middle finger on this wave, then comb down in the opposite direction to the position of the first dip, as in Fig. 25.

Great care must be taken to prevent too much hair being combed to the

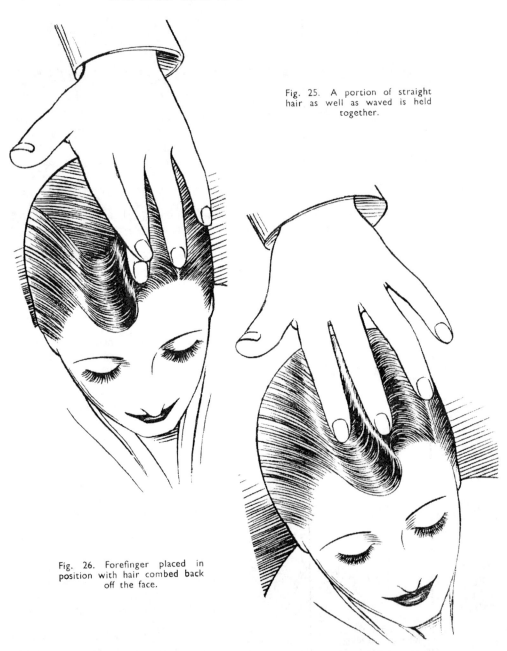

Fig. 25. A portion of straight hair as well as waved is held together.

Fig. 26. Forefinger placed in position with hair combed back off the face.

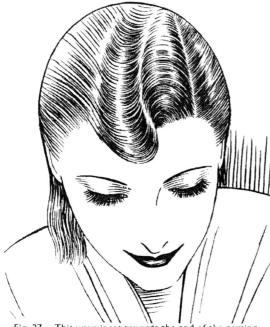

Fig. 27.   This wave is set towards the end of the parting.

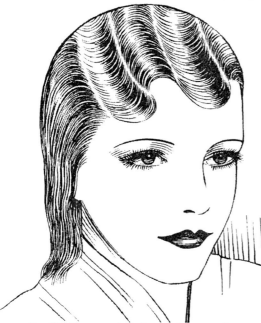

Fig. 28.   The second dip is placed on temple.

front; only the hair nearest the hair-line must be brought to the dip. Place the fore-finger in position on this dip and hold firmly, then comb the hair back off the face, as in the same illustration. Repeat this process farther up and along the head, slanting the wave until it disappears into the back of the parting; it is much easier for the student to do each wave separately than to place the waves in strips down, as the joining usually upsets the waves that have been done previously.

Joining The Waves

Experience has taught me that the student finds it difficult to join the waves; an explanation and an illustration (Fig. 25), will overcome this difficulty.

As you will observe, the middle finger is placed in such a position as to hold a portion of the hair already set, and a portion of the straight hair. Only the end of the comb is used in joining up, thus obviating the possibility of taking out the wave previously done. Comb the straight hair with the end portion of the comb tilted a little, and comb from close to the finger into the shape of the dip; then place the forefinger as shown in Fig. 26. The hair is now combed back.

Having carried out the first or peak wave successfully up to the crown, as in Fig. 27, continue with the second dip, which should be above the eyebrow, as in Fig. 28, and again comb all the hair back. The dip, now completed, should be on the hair line of the temple. The in-wave, previous to this dip, is the receding portion of the hair line, as before mentioned. The next in-wave, therefore, is the receding portion of the hair-line parallel with the eye, thus making the third dip the last wave, designated as the cheek wave, as in Figs. 29 and 30. The importance of the in-wave, level with the eye, cannot be over-

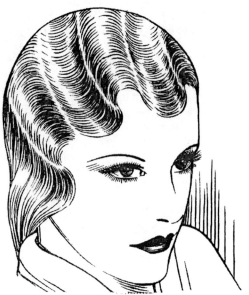

Fig. 29. The hair is combed well back on the in-wave prior to forming cheek wave.

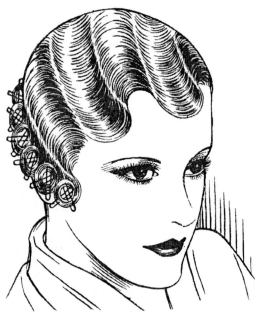

Fig. 30. Completed three dip dressing.

emphasised, because of its practicality.

This wave having been done in the correct way—that is, not allowing very much hair to be combed to the front and keeping all the waves parallel with the first one—the cheek wave has the precise amount of hair that the client needs, and not a tremendous thickness which becomes unruly after she has combed it herself.

If you believe these principles to be necessary to practical setting, you should not deviate from them. The dips must not become too slanted because this would bring the cheek wave behind the ear, instead of over it.

Correct and Incorrect Technique

As an example of the above-mentioned principles of my technique, compare the illustrations, Figs. 30 and 31. The latter, you will observe, is definitely against the hair line, and care must be taken to avoid this fault. The second dip is right on the eye and the cheek wave cannot therefore possibly be in the correct position.

Setting the Small Side of the Parting

Before completing the side referred to above, that is before attempting to complete the cheek wave by the curling—let us continue with the left side, which we will call the "small" side. But first I must emphasise most strongly this rule: "*The hair must be combed from the small side, towards the large side. The hair must never be combed from the large side to the small side.*" This rule must be remembered, because it will help with the following chapters.

Having combed the hair in the manner stated, continue by the upward movement from the parting. Place the middle finger down firmly on this movement, then comb

32

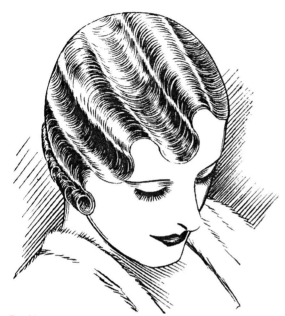

Fig. 31. Incorrect technique. Wave falling on to eye owing to the first dip being placed too low.

towards the crown, so that this wave will continue into the first dip wave on the large side. This will create a becoming slanting, waved back as in Fig. 34. Should horizontal waves be required at the back of the head however, the first in-wave on the small side is taken into the second dip, or temple wave, on the large side. In this case the waves on the small side will *not* be placed on such a slant as required for a diagonal back.

Placing the Curls

When you have completed the waving round the head, the next phase is curling. The easiest way to begin this is from the front of the small side, continuing up to the back of the ear, then proceeding with the other side, be-

the hair forward to form the first wave, or the first dip. This dip should be on the temple, level with the second dip on the other side, Fig. 32. The in-wave is therefore the same and so will be the cheek wave, as in Fig. 33.

There is an important point to mention here—the waves should be on a definite slant towards the crown, as this will help considerably when joining up the back waves.

Both sides having been completed, the next phase is the joining up of the back waves. The illustration in Fig. 34 will outline the necessary details. Having made note of my rule concerning the hair being combed from the small side to the large, we will continue with the in-wave level with the eye on the small side, and gradually slope upwards

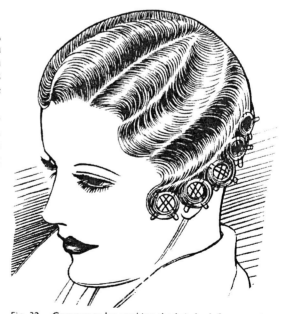

Fig. 32. Commence by combing the hair back from parting.

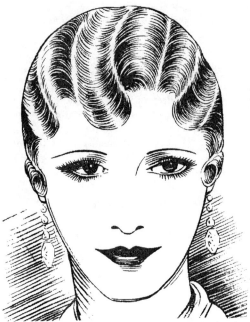

Fig. 33. Showing the temple waves level on both sides, the in-waves and cheek waves likewise.

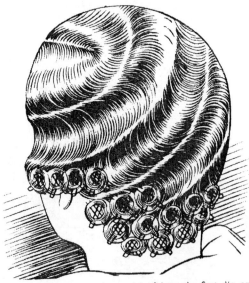

Fig. 34. The in-wave is continued into the first dip on large side.

ginning at the back of the ear and continuing to the front. This method makes the work much more simplified. The curling, as stated in the chapter "Hair Curling," must be carried right up to the ridge of the wave; if this is not done, the curls will drop and become lank, instead of having that springiness which is the essence of durability and which is so essential. There should never be fewer than four curls over each ear; if there are fewer the top of the ear will show; these curls are pinned to each other, so that they all hold each other in position when placed *en pli*. The illustrations show the hair pins crossed over. They can be inserted as shown on Fig. 2.

The Technique of Water-Waving

Three Dip Mode

One of the most practical coiffures asked for in a saloon that caters for a medium-class clientele is the "Three Dip" style, as shown in the illustration, Fig. 35. This design may seem to be similar to the design in Fig. 33, for technical details of the hair line are the same; the difference is this: that instead of the waves being set parallel with the parting, they are set in a much more circular position. The first wave looses itself into the parting, so that the first in-wave is brought round the crown and set into the first wave on the small side. This first wave on the small side is, therefore, in the same position as the second dip on the large side.

It cannot be emphasised too strongly that the hair must not on any account be brought to the front; only the hair that grows near the hair line must be set to form the dips.

Remember always that to carry out these designs successfully the correct technique must be adopted. A client will comb her hair off the face, and by so doing, she will comb the waves in accordance with the way the hair has been set. The general technical principle of this design, is to be sure that the first dip is as close up to the centre peak as possible; otherwise the dip will be far too low, and the waves for the temple and cheek wave will not fall into the correct technical position.

The dressing-out of the three-dip mode is as follows. Comb the hair right off the face and push forward; make sure that the dips are not too heavy. Should a deeper wave be necessary, then spray the hair with lotion or water, replace the veil and pinch up the ridges, beginning from the bottom wave.

Two Dip Mode

Here we have practical hair styles that are very effective if carried out correctly. The two dip mode was a fashionable style for many years among the smartest and most exclusive Mayfair clientele. I have found that the majority of women can carry this style, but I believe that a great number of hairdressers are doubtful about the correct procedure of this very attractive, artistic and practical design.

The individuality of this coiffure depends on its naturalness as well as its adaptability. With this dressing a client can comb her hair quite freely without fear that the waves will not respond to the combing.

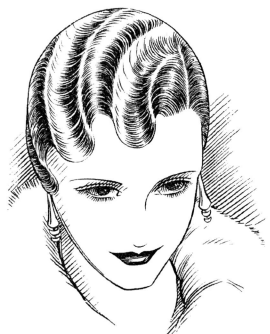

Fig. 35. Waves set in circular position. The first wave is lost in the parting.

To help you to produce something artistic, distinctive, and practical, I am including the accompanying sketches showing the two dip mode that will meet the demands of women who desire a practical and becoming Water-wave.

By having only the two waves—that is, the temple and the cheek wave—it reveals practically the entire hair line. Fig. 36 clearly shows that the hair is taken right back, and only the front hair is moulded into shape for the temple dip. When this wave is moulded into expression the in-wave is taken right back, to prevent any heaviness from falling on to the cheek wave. Skilful work is impossible unless the in-wave is in the correct position—level with the eye.

With this style of hair-dress the small side can be varied into different designs. Two waves on the small side, as in Fig. 32, can be done to look effective, but care must be taken in the first movement.

To produce the most effective result, the hair must be taken as far back as possible nearest the parting to have the same

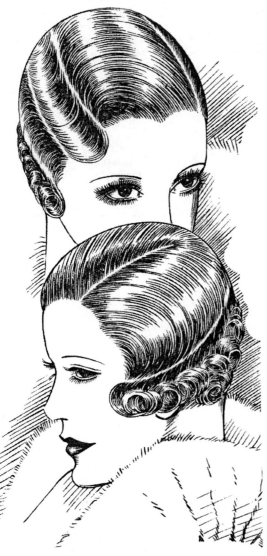

effect as the large side. The first ridge on the small side is taken to the end of the parting; the in-wave is therefore set into the temple wave on the large side.

Varying the Design of the Small Side

A delightful variation of the small side that will harmonise attractively with the large side of the two dip coiffure is the design illustrated in Fig. 37. This shows a dressing that is the true elegance of hair artistry. The graceful movement of the swathed expression may seem to be over-emphasised, but I can assure readers that enormous possibilities are at their disposal if they can justify the demands of these practical coiffures. Even if some of these designs may seem to be far-fetched they are practical, and sooner or later you may be called upon to carry them out.

The reason for including this design (Fig. 37), is to show and explain that sleekness in coiffure-arrangement can be simple yet original. There are a number of women who prefer a very low parting with the two dip mode. The hair taken back on the small side would, therefore, look very effective.

Another pleasing yet simple design for the small side, which harmonises with the two dip coiffure, is the one illustrated in Fig. 38. The first wave, in this instance, is moulded into a downward movement, yet the hair is kept off the face. Should the hair not be taken off the face, then a straight appearance would follow, which would not reveal the artistic line that is necessary for successful setting.

Fig. 36 (top). The hair is swept right back to prevent any heaviness on the dip.

Fig. 37. An artistic expression of sleekness.

Two-wave Coiffure

Another two-wave coiffure I am presenting may seem at first to be very simple to carry out, but despite its apparent simplicity the correct technique must be used. Fig. 39 shows that the dip is higher than the previous illustration relating to the two dip mode. Half the ear in Fig. 39 is clearly shown, and the hair at the end of the wave is curled. Although I am not including an illustration for the small side of this coiffure, you will not find it difficult to do.

By covering up the dip, leaving only the bottom wave, you will observe the position of the wave required for the small side. In joining up the back waves, the eye-level in-wave of the large side is continued into the first wave of the small side.

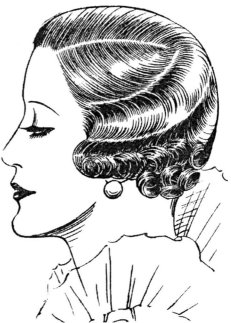

Fig. 38. Showing the first movement, a downward wave from the parting.

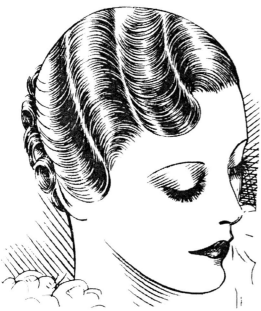

Fig. 39. Showing wave over half the ear, with curls at the back.

Fig. 40 presents the small side design of a two dip mode, but the waves are brought still higher to show the whole of the ear; yet the correct technique is applied. The waves in this case are set almost oblique. The hair must be placed in the correct position before setting—that is, it must be combed right across from the small side. The upward wave over the ear on the small side is continued up and set into the dip on the large side. In carrying out this design, find the correct length of hair that will be required for the curls by combing from the small side into the position where the curls will be in the completed coiffure, as shown in Fig. 41. The hair must be well tapered to ensure easy manipulation. In preparing the correct length for this coiffure, comb all

37

the hair in position—that is, for a left side parting comb into position as shown in the completed dressing. By observing this principle the correct length can easily be prepared for the curls.

The dressing-out of this coiffure is a simple one. Comb the hair right through the waves and curls, spray brilliantine, replace the waves in position, and dress the curls. Should the waves not be as deep as you would like them, then spray a little setting lotion or water, replace the net and pinch up, drying with a hand dryer. The bottom wave is the first wave to be redried.

Uniformity in coiffure designs is now a thing of the past. It has been replaced with designs of individuality and interpreted for the consideration of mode expres-

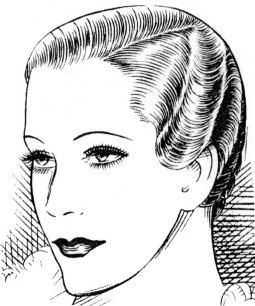

Fig. 40. The first movement is combed right back from the parting.

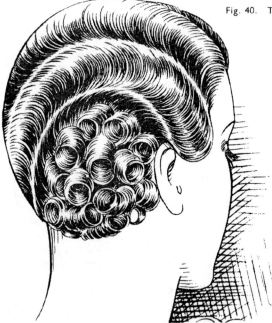

Fig. 41. The hair is combed from the small side to the large side with the ends placed in curls.

sion. An example of coiffure arrangement is explained in the accompanying illustration. Fig. 42. This mode is designed to abandon the once-prevailing uniformity.

The swathed effect gives it that charm of distinction.

This design is attractive for the woman with a shingle, although it is very becoming with curls low at the nape. It also has a tendency to lengthen the shape of a short head. This swathed movement must be combed from the small side—that is, from the side of the parting—to the large side, as explained on page 33.

The easiest way to carry out the swathed back is on the two dip mode, Fig. 36. After completing the *mis-en-pli* on both sides, begin a wave near the crown on the large side so that this wave is completed into the cheek wave on the small side, as in Fig. 42. To avoid having an abundance of unwanted hair when completed, the hair should be tapered after it has been combed, and replaced in position as is necessary for the completed coiffure. The graduation in the taper will necessitate the hair being longer at the beginning of the swathe than where the swathe ends. This important tapering, in conjunction with the swathed design, will give that added elegance to the deportment of a well-dressed woman.

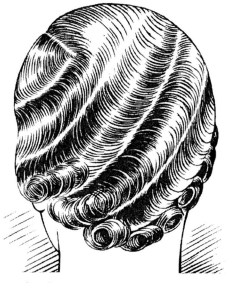

Fig. 42. Showing waves on an extreme slant. Hair *must* be combed from small side to the large side before making pli.

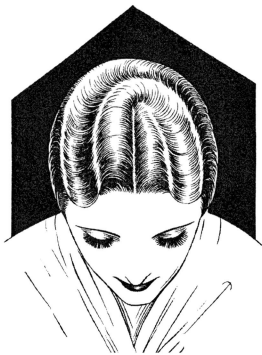

Fig. 43. Note the first ridge on the right side continued to end of parting.

Centre Parting

You have probably been asked by clients on many occasions: "Do you think a centre parting will suit me?" A definite answer will give the discriminating woman the impression that she is being attended to by a hairdresser who is also an artist. The client's object in suggesting a centre parting is because she thinks her looks will be improved, but before deciding on this change she wants the hairdresser's advice.

A centre parting tends to alter the whole appearance; it can have the effect of broadening or lengthening the face. I do not advise the introduction of a centre parting to a woman with a very high forehead.

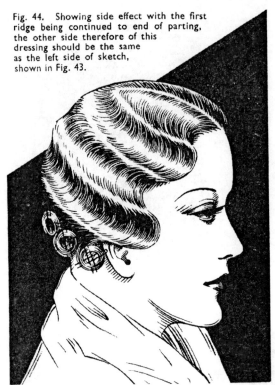

Fig. 44. Showing side effect with the first ridge being continued to end of parting, the other side therefore of this dressing should be the same as the left side of sketch, shown in Fig. 43.

A great number of outstanding coiffures can be achieved with a centre parting and can be made into a number of pleasing and appealing designs. The illustrations in Figs. 43 and 44 show practical designs and explain correct technique. Fig. 44 favours two waves on each side of the parting and Fig. 43 explains the movements for joining the waves at the crown. In the latter illustration you will observe that the dips are exactly in the same position, but a wave on one side near the crown is moved slightly inwards to allow the first in-wave on one side to continue into the first dip on the other side, the first in-wave on one side losing itself in the parting, as indicated in the illustration.

Pompadour

There are a number of styles that cannot be practised very frequently because they are seldom demanded. For this reason I say, most strongly, that you must not wait until a client asks for a certain style, and then, when you begin to do it, practise at the same time. Allocate a little time to the practising of the various coiffures that may be asked for, even if they do not include the styles of the present mode.

A majority of our clients probably favour the parting head-dress; only a very small group favour the hair combed over into pompadour style. The hair combed right back can be varied into different designs. The full pompadour is the style taken straight back as in Fig. 45. The semi-pompadour has a dip on one side as in Fig. 46, and the two-dip-pompadour, as in Fig. 47, is a dressing which is very difficult to carry out, and one that requires a great deal of practice.

The Full Pompadour. Fig. 45.

To follow the movements very carefully, turn the sketch upside down; you will then be able to see and follow the best method to adopt. The hair is combed perfectly flat and thoroughly wetted with setting lotion; a little heavy setting lotion will help to keep the hair in position. To begin, comb the hair to the right or left (it does not make any difference, but in this case you will find it easier to follow the sketch) in a right circular movement beginning in the centre and forming a circular effect towards the hair line.

The next wave is now combed towards the left and continued to the front of the left ear as shown in Fig. 48. The up-wave over the left ear is continued in a circular movement towards the front of the right ear, so that a definite wave is shown on both sides alike. The up-wave over the ear on the right side is continued round, so that the wave falls behind the left ear. The waves are continued to the nape of the neck and finished off in curls; should the hair be long, it is waved as far as the nape.

The Semi or Broken Pompadour. Fig. 46.

This dressing is rather more difficult than the Pompadour, and gives the student a little trouble to produce. Although this style is not very common nowadays, all hairdressers should know how to achieve it. The most difficult part of all is to make the waves fall precisely in the right position on the forehead, temples and cheek.

To prepare for this style, the hair must be well-saturated with lotion to avoid any unwanted divisions. The hair should be combed a little towards the side that requires the dip. In the illustration, it favours a right side dip with a cheek wave, but it can also be waved obliquely over the ears. As for the pompadour, by turning the sketch upside down, you will notice that the hair has been combed towards the left, beginning in the centre. Place your middle finger firmly on this impression and comb towards the right, still in the centre. Continue down towards the dip. The dip *must* be close up to the centre or peak, otherwise it will be impossible to obtain three waves as illustrated.

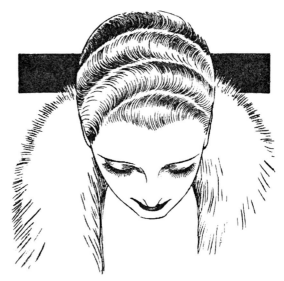

Fig. 45. To follow the movements correctly, turn this dressing upside down, commencing in the centre.

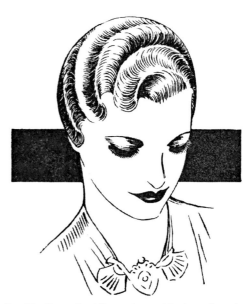

Fig. 46. For a Semi-Pompadour with three dips, the first dip must commence near the centre or peak.

41

Double Dip Pompadour. Fig. 47.

I know that this dressing will present great difficulty in its manipulation. It is not practised very much to-day, but this book would be incomplete without reference to it. The enterprising hairdresser should not neglect this style because it is difficult.

And the greatest difficulty in carrying out the double dip pompadour is avoiding the possibility of a slight parting in the centre. Again, the easiest method is to turn the sketch upside down. The wave in the centre *must* be done first; then place the dips as near to the peak or centre as possible, making perfectly sure that the dips are level on both sides. Once the front dips are completed, continue the waves, preferably off the face, exposing the ears.

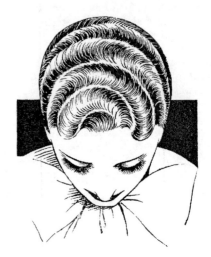

Fig. 47. Commence the first wave in the centre. The first dips should be as near the centre or peak as possible.

The up-wave below the first dip is continued round the head in a circular position to the temple of the left side; this should be level with a temple wave on the other side which has not yet been formed. The up-wave below the temple wave of the left side is now continued round to the temple of the right side, as shown in the illustration. When these waves are continued, the cheek wave will automatically fall into the correct position. Should the hair be short, the cheek wave can be curled; if long, then make a complete wave over the ear, curling the extreme ends. Should the client request a semi-pompadour with two waves showing the ears or part of the ears, the dressing would be similar to the two-dip in Fig. 39. This design is popular and practical.

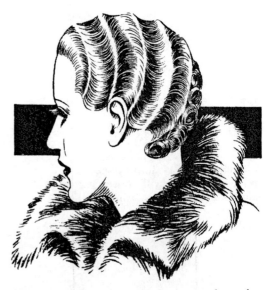

Fig. 48. Full Pompadour. Waves placed in front of ear on both sides.

CHAPTER SEVEN

Water-waving with Setting Combs

There is usually a controversy about the method of Water-waving with setting combs. Some masters do not accept their use as a practical method of setting the hair. When Marcel waving was the vogue, and only women with naturally wavy or permanently waved hair visited the hairdresser for setting, it was not essential for the hairdresser to use setting combs. Nowadays, with permanent waving having almost replaced Marcel waving, Water-waving is in greatest demand.

When a permanent wave has grown out, women still require their hair Water-waved, although their hair is straight. This is one of the occasions when setting combs should be used. Although I do not advocate the use of setting combs on all types of hair, there are, of course, many occasions when I do consider their use necessary to assist in strengthening the wave. The use of setting combs need not be confined to straight hair only. They can be used on all types of hair provided they are used correctly.

Students must be familiar with the use of combs for Water-waving, whether they agree with their use or not. Even among the masters of Water-waving, there are different opinions about this method of setting the hair; nevertheless, it is a recognised fact that satisfactory results can be obtained with the use of setting combs, provided they are correctly placed in the waves. It is well known that some high-class establishments are continually using these combs; and in some places, when they are not used, clients demand them because they believe that the waves last much longer.

It may be of interest to the reader if I mention a few of the early efforts to carry out a Water-wave with setting combs. When hairdressers were acknowledged as expert Marcel wavers, and when they were not prepared for the growing demand for Water-waving, they developed their own methods; with the use of setting combs they made an impression of a wave and then inserted a comb; made another impression and inserted another comb, and so on. This method was undoubtedly the only one known to them. Nevertheless, they had water-waved their clients' hair.

This system compares very unfavourably with to-day's method. Modern demands have given hairdressers an opportunity to discard those early efforts which they now know to be impractical. Nowadays, the straightest of hair can be water-waved, and the procedure is the same as that of ordinary water waving without the use of setting combs. With the introduction of heavier types of setting lotion, water-waving is much more simplified than it was in the earlier days. The heavier type of lotion helps to hold the hair in position, thus enabling the operator to place the entire hair in pli before using the setting combs.

43

It is necessary to have about 20 to 25 flexible setting combs. Some of these can be broken in two, as small combs are essential for joining up the setting when space does not allow for a full-size comb.

When setting a straight head of hair certain definite rules and principles must be adopted; one of the most important is that the hair must be kept smoothly combed out all the time, and must have sufficient moisture to make it pliable. Remember always that the hair cannot be pliable unless it is thoroughly saturated. Smooth setting and not deep setting is essential, when setting combs are to be used. Deep setting would mean that the hair nearest the scalp might not be in the same position as the waved hair on top, thus preventing the setting comb from making a firm foundation as it does when the hair is set smoothly and evenly.

Assuming that we are carrying out a dressing favouring the three dip mode with curls on the cheek wave; having placed the hair in pli correctly, and before the curls are completed, continue as follows:—

The first setting comb must be inserted on the lowest wave—the in-wave as illustrated in Fig. 49.—so that when completed the wave holds the top hair in position. Should you begin with the first dip, then you will probably upset the position of the lower waves. Before inserting the comb, hold in position as in Fig. 49. (note that the comb is straightened), insert towards the left, this being the position of the wave. The next comb is therefore pushed up towards the right, and so on.

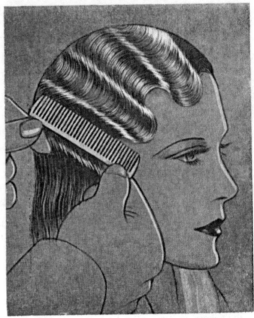

Fig. 49. Place the first Setting Comb in the in-wave level with the eye.

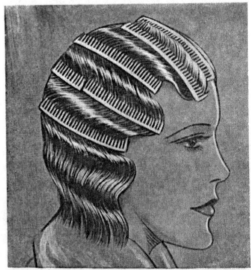

Fig. 50. Note that the combs on the first dip are interlaced but not locked together.

WATER-WAVING WITH SETTING COMBS

It is not necessary to follow the same ridge all round the head to prevent the top hair being upset, but the combs can be placed one above the other in sections. They need not be pushed up until all are inserted, and the curls on the sides and back completed. Should the hair be very straight, and a good impression needed, place a setting comb facing the first comb in the first dip. The illustration in Fig. 50 clearly shows this comb in the completed position, but great care must be taken not to lock the teeth of the combs together, as this would form a hard and ugly ridge. The comb facing should be placed in such a position to allow the hair near the parting to obtain a clearer and more definite shape of a wave.

Having completed the entire head, setting combs and curls, the hair is now ready for drying; but before doing so, cover the head with a water-waving net, pinned fairly tightly. The waves can be pushed up slightly, beginning at the bottom wave.

Do not forget to insert a piece of cotton wool under the cheek wave to prevent the heat of the pins from touching the face.

When the hair has been thoroughly dried, and the combs and pins removed, the hair must be combed through thoroughly to take away the heaviness of the ridge and comb marks.

The heavier type of setting lotion has a tendency to dry hard, but as soon as the hair is combed the waves become softer. After the hair has been carefully combed and the curls dressed out, spray with a little water or setting lotion. Replace the net and finish off with a hand dryer, pinching up the waves, beginning on the bottom wave and gradually pinching up each ridge.

By following the instructions and illustrations submitted, and with a little practice, the student should have additional confidence in the manipulation of setting combs. These combs, however, should not be used continuously, but only on difficult heads such as those with straight hair, or on hair that has been dyed or on coarse hair.

It is not advisable to use setting combs on hair that has been over-bleached, as this will make the ridges of the waves have an exceptionally hard and unnatural appearance. A good spirit setting lotion is sufficient to enable one to water-wave bleached hair successfully because of its pliability. Practice will tell which type of hair is most suitable for comb setting.

CHAPTER EIGHT

Drying the Hair after Water-Waving

There is a perfectly logical reason why a few lines on the subject of hair drying are introduced here. The reason is, that on numerous occasions I have seen a beautiful *mis-en-pli* spoilt through not drying the hair correctly. Not so very long ago, it was the practise for a hairdresser to hold a hand dryer over the hair after it had been set, and push up the waves until dry. This procedure usually made the hair fluffy, but the present mode of sleekness and softness prevents the hair from being dried in this manner. The potentialities of the process of hood drying eliminates the fluffiness produced by hand drying. It is impossible to dry the hair by hand satisfactorily in some of the designs submitted in this publication, especially those with sleek dressings and curled fronts. By allowing the hair to dry in the same position as it is set, the result will obviously be much more satisfactory and the curls can be dressed according to the position of the first "pli." The process of such drying is the same as when attending to postiche. The hair is put in "pli," placed in an oven until dry, dressed out again and placed in the oven for another period. The drying of to-day is therefore based upon the principles adopted for postiche. As soon as the hair is set and the net placed over, not too tightly, pinch the waves, commencing at the bottom wave. By commencing at the bottom, the upsetting of the other waves is overcome. Should you start at the top, and the first wave is pushed up, the other waves are automatically pulled out of position. Before placing the hood over the hair, place a piece of cotton wool under the net and over the ears to prevent them getting hot. The cotton wool also prevents the pins from touching the ears or the face.

Hair Must be Combed through after Drying

There are a great number of women who cannot comb their hair properly, irrespective of how it has been set. Therefore it is important when doing a practical design, to ascertain the exact way the client combs her hair. Having set the hair in the style the client wishes and having thoroughly dried it, remove the pins and net, and comb the hair right through. I do not mean comb each wave separately as if you are setting the hair, but with one swoop right through the hair. I know that some readers will imagine that this will spoil the effect; on the contrary, it will give an added effect to the whole dressing. When the waves have ultimately been recombed into position and the curls combed separately with the aid of a tail comb, the net can be replaced, and the hair sprayed with setting lotion or water, so that it is just slightly damp. Pinch each wave separately, commencing as outlined above, by starting at the bottom wave. This extra pinching up, gives that added tightness and durability, deepens the waves and gives a much more compact and lasting effect. The combing through, after the hair has been dried, does not apply to every style, but only to practical waved styles for everyday wear. It would be futile to comb the hair through and re-comb the curls of coiffures that have been specially placed in "pli" for specific styles.

46

CHAPTER NINE

Styling Ahead

FOLLOWING a previous chapter on practical water-waving, this chapter will help the enthusiastic hairdresser to improve his knowledge of hair designing.

Many years of teaching have convinced me that the art and practice of water-waving is the essential foundation of successful styling. Hairdressing to-day calls for intricate styling which can be achieved only by skilful work. This art enables us to present a good shape and an artistic line.

Hairdressing can be classified according to the clientele. Some establishments cater only for the hard, solid type of work—deep waves and curls; two or three waves close to the face. Other saloons, especially those in Mayfair, incorporate very few waved styles in their hair designing. The introduction of new hair styles in the former establishment is not always easy, but to become an artistic stylist you must constantly vary your work and use your imagination to the full. Your clients, if properly educated by you, will appreciate this variation.

A good conscientious waver can easily become a good stylist. Almost all styles shown in this book up to now are not only of a practical, everyday nature, but are also styles that you will be constantly asked to carry out. Having studied and practised the basic principles of Practical Water-waving you can then learn elaborate hair styling.

CHAPTER TEN

The Definition of Beauty

A CORRECT definition of beauty is rather difficult to give because of the variety of causes and component parts which help to make a complete picture. Hair dressed correctly and in proper proportion helps to produce perfect beauty. This perfection is embodied in the woman whose temperament and personality express the complete ensemble. A combination of these qualities would show us the highest type of beauty—a type difficult to attain, because each of these qualities must be perfect in itself to form a completely beautiful whole. Beautiful hair predominates in making up beauty, and, in designing a hair style, the personality of the woman *must* therefore be considered.

How often do we wonder what it is that makes a woman's head so dignified or stylish, when, in fact, it is simply that the particular style suits her? There might be a hundred different modifications of the various styles, with an analysis of the meaning and expression of each one—the merry and the melancholy, the sophisticated and the timid, the saintly and the coquettish, the practical and the poetical, each finding a picture of her particular style. The hairdresser must guard against stumbling ignorantly and unconsciously upon a style which is entirely out of harmony with the lady's character.

Science and Art might well combine to give it some comprehensible system. The variation of present-day modes differ with individuals. Some dressings are low, others high as in Edwardian styles, but the dictates of fashion, as in everything else, simplicity in the arrangement, and grace in the direction of the lines, are the chief points to be considered. In or out of fashion, curls are pre-eminently attractive and becoming. Few faces are beautiful enough to be without them, although in some cases, sleek, artistic movements can be equally becoming, should they harmonise with the personality of the wearer.

The most beautiful women are said to be those with oval faces. Art teaches us how to produce the effect of an oval, even when the shape does not actually exist, but certain rules must be respected. For instance, never allow the head to look too large; never allow too much hair on the neck unless the design is proportioned accordingly. If the lady is very tall avoid piling the hair too high, and, if she is short, avoid any bulkiness about the neck or head; in fact, study proportion.

A real artist always considers proportion and studies what is appropriate.

The variety of opinions on beauty differ; one may admire the tall and graceful, another the short and petite, but never copy a hair style, no matter how fashionable it may be, unless you are certain that the individual is the right type to wear it. That is what I mean by "appropriate."

48

CHAPTER ELEVEN

Direction of Lines

The accompanying illustrations, Fig. 51, will help the student to understand and follow the correct direction of the line of a hair-style design. These principles are important, but, of course, modifications can be made.

If the hair is properly shaped it forms an attractive contour of its own. This should be emphasised, as many hair designs have been spoiled by not following the correct line of direction. The principles for creating width in a horizontal position, and an elongated effect with the diagonal and vertical line, must be clearly understood, for not only does the direction of line apply to waving but also to combing.

The sketches here will help the untrained eye to achieve accuracy in shape and individuality in design.

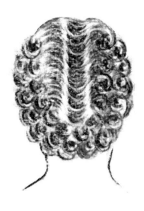 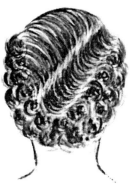 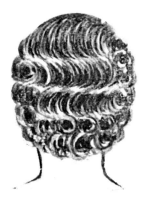

Vertical   Diagonal   Horizontal.

Fig. 51.

Twelve Basic Principles

THIS chapter gives the detailed information that is so important. It will serve as a reference and a supplementary text, and is helped by sketches which are easy to follow.

A sound scientific foundation, which all hairdressers should endeavour to achieve, is the basis for creating hair styles.

The twelve basic principles hold the answers to many problems that arise daily in the saloon. As each chapter is studied you will eventually refer to these illustrations to help you to carry out certain styles, for they reflect the hair fashions that are most in demand. To achieve the best result each basic principle should be studied, practised, and adapted; and when you have mastered it, try to incorporate other designs to that movement. You will be able to adapt these movements to any hair style you see, and by doing so, you will in time find also that you can create your own designs.

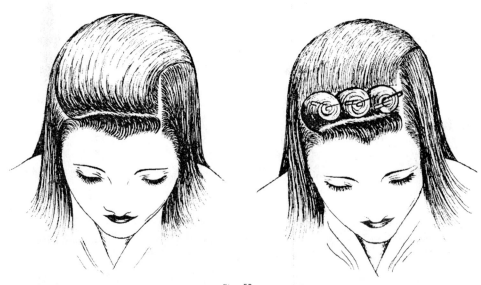

Fig. 52.
Basic No. 1.

TWELVE BASIC PRINCIPLES

Basic No. 1, Fig. 52.

This movement should be the first method to study for styling. It incorporates your training in water-waving, and although the parting in the illustration shows a left side parting, the practice of movements for the right side is the same.

Observe the completed dressing Fig. 53. Basic No. 1. You will notice this is a large swirl, made from the three curls. Should the style necessitate separate curls, then each curl can be back-combed to create a fuller effect. The distance from the hair line to the crest of the wave should not be too wide, as this ridge helps to make the front swirl stand more upright. The further the crest of the wave is made from the hair line the more likely the swirl is to fall back, as the wave itself acts as a foundation.

To obtain the correct effect, the most important rule to remember is to comb the hair slightly towards the parting, and make the crest in an absolutely horizontal line. Having completed this movement, select the width of hair required for the curls by placing the point of the tail comb directly through the

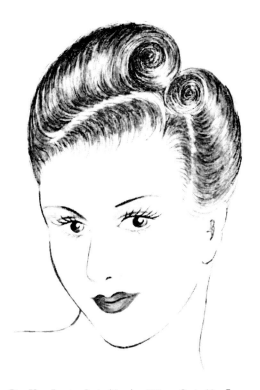

Fig. 53. *Front.* Basic No. 1. *Sides.* Basic No. 7.

hair on to the scalp. By doing this a clean parting is ensured. The first curl to pin is the one nearest to the parting, and the pin of the second curl should penetrate through to the first curl and make both curls more secure. The third curl should be a larger movement which will make the dressing-out easier because of the overlapping of the swirl. When a tight, small curl is made, a large movement is difficult to obtain as the smallness of the circumference of the curl will fall in a wave. A further row of curls, going in the same direction, can be made for a swirl, should a larger movement be required. Two rows of curls are also essential when the hair is not too curly. A setting comb can be placed just under the crest to keep the wave in position while curling, or to accentuate the crest should the hair have very little wave in it.

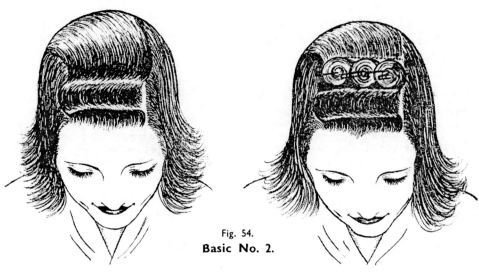

Fig. 54.
Basic No. 2.

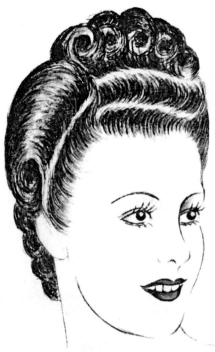

Basic No. 2. Fig. 54.

This design is also for a swirled effect, but with a completed wave. As in Basic 1, the hair is combed slightly towards the parting, then a complete wave is made. In this case the first curl to be pinned is the one farthest from the parting. During the process of water-waving the hair must always be kept smoothly combed out.

Fig. 55.
Front. Basic No. 2.
Sides. Basic No. 8.

52

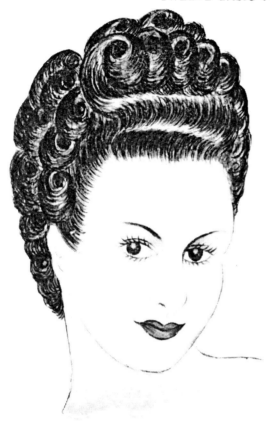

Fig. 56. Basic No. 2. Showing right side parting. *Sides.* Basic No. 8

Basic No. 3. Fig. 57.

The pli for the frontal effect having been completed, the side movement essential to learn is one which will harmonise with the swirled design. First make a parting to the back of the ear as shown in the illustration. Then make an upward movement close to the hair line, and with the point of the tail comb divide the hair so that you have a clean parting. The curl is not placed on its own base, but swirled up; this position simplifies the dressing-out. The remaining hair should be curled in position as in Basic 10.

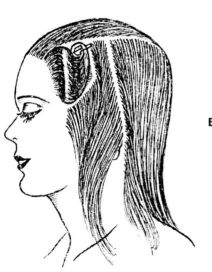

Fig. 57.

Basic No. 3.

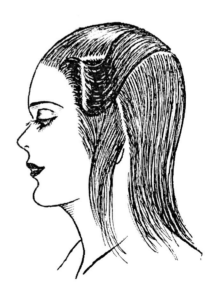

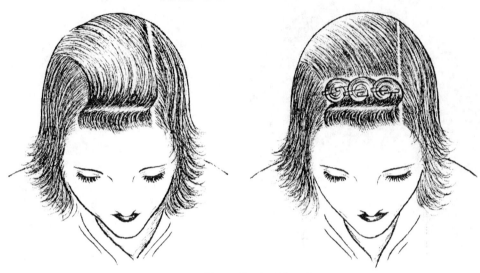

Fig. 58.   **Basic No. 4.**

Basic No. 4. Fig. 58.

The method of preparation is the opposite to that of Basic 1: instead of combing the first movement towards the parting, the first movement of Basic 4 is combed the opposite way. The first curl to be pinned is the one farthest from the parting, so that the last curl could have a longer stem for an overlapping movement as shown on the basic chart.

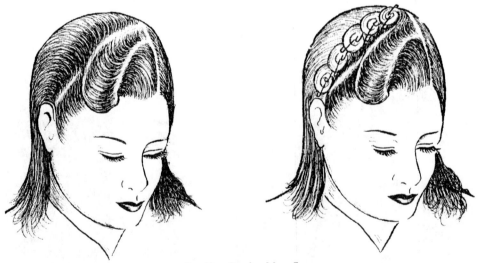

Fig. 59.   **Basic No. 5.**

54

TWELVE BASIC PRINCIPLES

Basic No. 5. Fig. 59.

Although this is a very practical design it can be quite effective. It is capable of considerable variation. Preliminary tapering is a very important point that must be considered for any of the designs I have included, but particularly so for this style as it lends itself to a soft fluffy effect. An extra row of curls going in the opposite direction will give the dressing a fuller design. This design creates height and is very effective in enhancing the appearance of a woman with a round face.

Basic No. 6. Fig. 60.

The introduction of anything new always makes certain people apprehensive. If your client is a very conservative type, used to one style only, a new style should be presented as an easy style. Basic No. 6 is a simple mode with which to make a change-over. It is quite in keeping with present-day fashion. It has an artistic line, and when properly combed-out presents a good shape. A successful dressing depends on the skilful manner in which the wave is placed. As in previous designs, the position of the first movement is the most important one. Make absolutely certain that this first movement is combed towards the parting, irrespective of which side the parting is. Should the hair not respond to a good crest because of its lack of curl or wave, then place a setting comb under the crest. This comb can remain in during the drying period. The *CC* curls as shown should be close to the crest, which will improve the shape when dressed out. A second row of *CC* curls is advisable, to obtain a larger movement and a more solid dressing. The first curl to be done is the one nearest the parting. Special care is needed with the last curl, as you will see that this one is not pinned on its own base, but swirled upwards to give a longer movement, which obviates the possibility of another wave appearing in the large swirl.

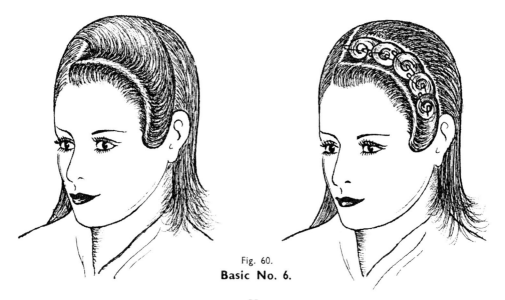

Fig. 60.
Basic No. 6.

55

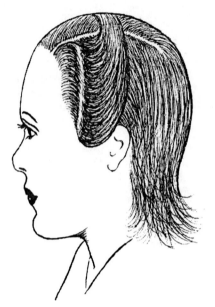
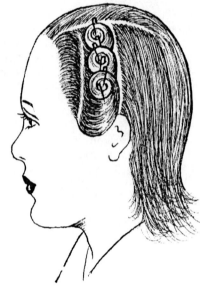

Fig. 61. **Basic No. 7.**

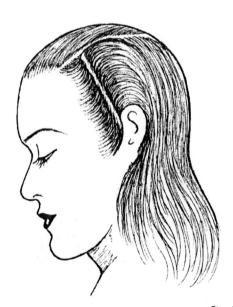
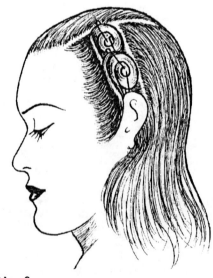

Fig. 62. **Basic No. 8.**

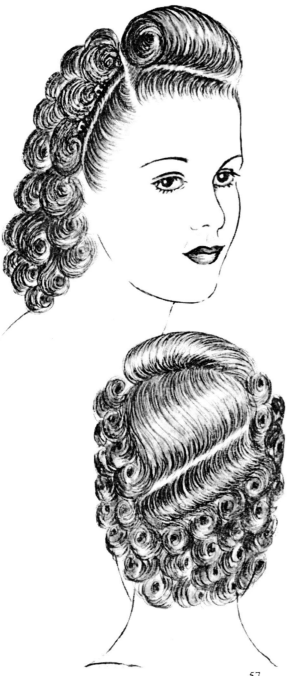

Basic No. 7. Fig. 61.

The technique for the small side of a swirled dressing is the same as that for the large side. The most important points to remember are: the hair should be well combed up from the hair line, and the crest not too far away. The first curl to be pinned is the one nearest the parting, and it should be as close to the parting as possible. The closer together the first curls are, the higher the swirls can be dressed, and the smarter the appearance of the whole effect. On both sides the last curl is done with a decidedly longer movement.

Basic No. 8. Fig. 62.

Unique effects in coiffure arrangements can easily be achieved if the art and technique are known. The arrangement of a distinctive style depends upon the artistic mind. Basic No. 8 defines that interpretation of artistic conception. The side arrangement shown can be adapted to many frontal designs. The important point to follow is the definite down movement when making the first wave. Although some of these basic drawings show the side effects only, the top dressing should always be done before the sides.

Fig. 63.

Front. Basic No. 1.
Back. Basic No. 12.
Sides. Basic No. 8.

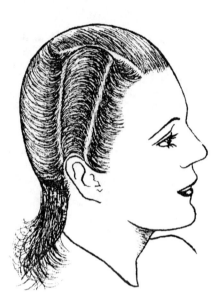
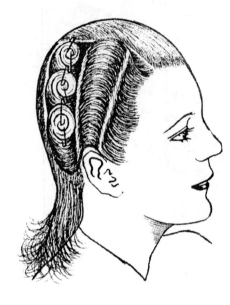

Fig. 64.
Basic No. 9.

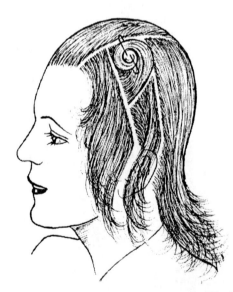
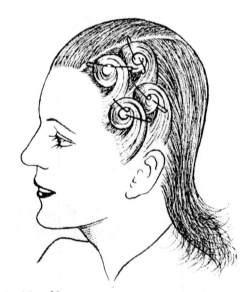

Fig. 66. **Basic No. 10.**

TWELVE BASIC PRINCIPLES

Basic No. 9. Fig. 64.

Women always look forward to something new. Their charm depends largely upon the graceful coiffures which the hairdresser presents. Basic No. 9 is not a complicated design. It is practical and one that the client can comb herself, and yet when properly arranged it can be varied to pleasing and artistic positions. I need not elaborate upon the procedure of the pli; the illustration clearly explains the movements.

Basic No. 10. Fig. 66.

Hair styling fundamentals are based on the theory of balanced lines. Obviously it is impossible in this limited space to sketch all basic principles for to-day's fashion, but those which I am including are the simple movements which you can master and which will enable you to improve and vary your styles.

Basic No. 10 is the important foundation of good artistic hair styling, and I recommend you to study and practise the making of swirl curls to absolute perfection. Perfect swirl curls will give you the enthusiasm for creative hair designing. The beauty of a nice

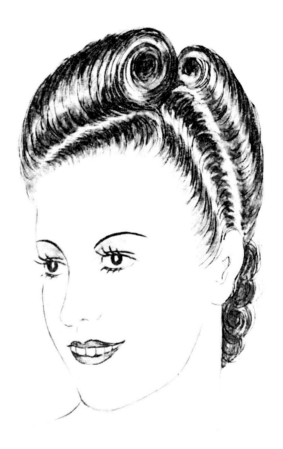

Fig. 65. *Front.* Basic No. 1. *Sides.* Basic No. 9.

curl depends upon its shape and roundness. It is particularly important for you to study the making of the partings or divisions to obtain the perfect swirl. Note carefully the illustration and observe the parting made on a slant. This slanting parting must be adhered to for the purpose of making swirled curls. If a straight or horizontal division were made there would be a break in the dressing, and should a large movement be desired, or if the curls were dressed out separately, they would flop and lose their shape.

59

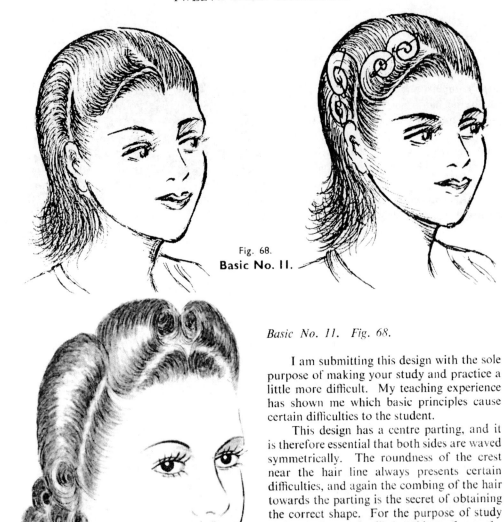

Fig. 68.
Basic No. II.

Basic No. 11. Fig. 68.

I am submitting this design with the sole purpose of making your study and practice a little more difficult. My teaching experience has shown me which basic principles cause certain difficulties to the student.

This design has a centre parting, and it is therefore essential that both sides are waved symmetrically. The roundness of the crest near the hair line always presents certain difficulties, and again the combing of the hair towards the parting is the secret of obtaining the correct shape. For the purpose of study and practice you will be able to learn the intricacy of C and CC curls when making waves. The basic chart illustrates an example of dignified lines of hair styling that will enable you to deal with all possible difficulties.

Fig. 69. *Sides.* Basic No. 5. *Front.* Basic No. II.

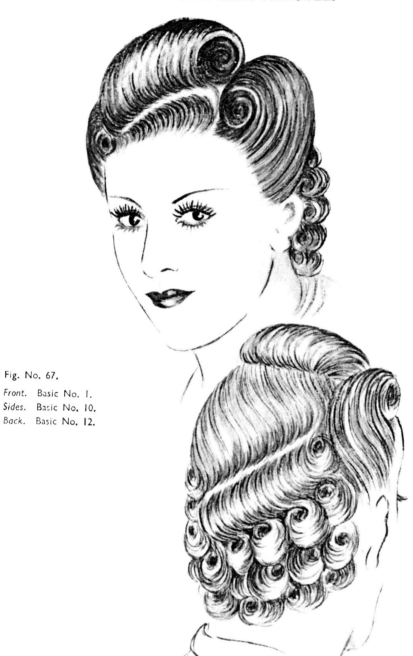

Fig. No. 67.

Front. Basic No. 1.
Sides. Basic No. 10.
Back. Basic No. 12.

Basic No. 12. Fig. 70.

When you carry out all these suggested designs the frontal effect should be done first. The sides should then be parted off and left to the last. The back dressing should be completed and then the sides put up. The reason for leaving the sides until last can be simply explained. Assuming for instance that you had completed the side movement Basic No. 10, you would find that the swirl curls would overlap the division and present difficulty in making the curls as shown in Basic 12. It is simpler and far more effective to complete the back dressing and then do the side movements. I fully appreciate that a student would find it very difficult to wave the sides without interfering with the back dressing. But if you place a towel over the hair that has been set, as in Fig. 71, you will not disturb it.

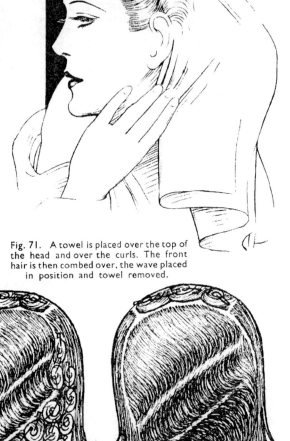

Fig. 71. A towel is placed over the top of the head and over the curls. The front hair is then combed over, the wave placed in position and towel removed.

The twelve modes that have been portrayed have been carefully selected for the student who wishes to improve his hairdressing technique. I am confident that by practising each basic movement you will steadily improve your knowledge. By combing and adapting styles, you will find that in time you can create for yourself an unending number of variations.

Fig. 70.
Basic No. 12.

62

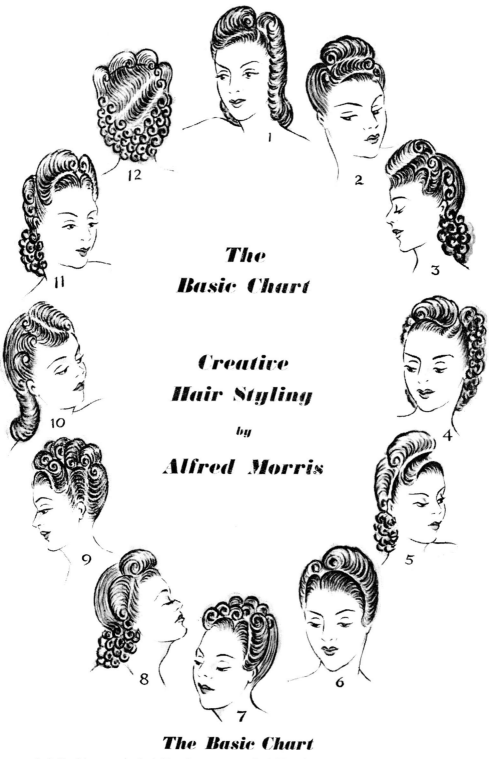

The
Basic Chart

Creative
Hair Styling

by

Alfred Morris

The Basic Chart

Basic No.		incorporating basic No.					
Basic No.	1	incorporating basic No.					8
,,	,,	2	,,	,,	,,	,,	10
,,	,,	3	,,	,,	,,	,,	5
,,	,,	4	,,	,,	,,	,,	8
,,	,,	5	,,	,,	,,	,,	2 and 8
,,	,,	6	,,	,,	,,	,,	7

Basic No.	7	incorporated basic No.				11 front
,,	,,	8	,,	,,	,,	,,	1
,,	,,	9	,,	,,	,,	3
,,	,,	10	,,	,,	Fig. 112 "Bang" design
,,	,,	11	,,	,,	basic Nos. 1 and 8
,,	,,	12	,,	,,	,, No. 10 sides

CHAPTER THIRTEEN

The Principles of Physiognomy

AN appreciation of women's features is the most important factor for the hairdresser, if he is to advise and create the *chic* coiffure that enhances feminine beauty. In other words, the perfection of hairdressing is the scientifically thought-out and well-groomed design, which does so much to achieve our modern idea of beauty.

Hair-styling is one of the fundamental principles of adornment for the completion of any woman's loveliness. Even the most ungainly head of hair can be transformed into an immaculate and becoming coiffure, and no woman should risk losing the prestige of that sense of personal importance and assurance which is achieved by having a coiffure suited to her appearance, personality and social background.

A well-groomed hair-style requires efficient manipulation; it is well to emphasise this, for efficiency may be interpreted as the main necessity for having a well-cared-for hair style. While the principles used for a style may be technical, they should not be incapable of self-manipulation, for a beautiful hair style can be practical although elaborate.

The secret of designing coiffures flattering to the individual lies primarily in suiting the hair fashion to the wearer, by careful study of the hair line, shape of profile, etc. Important rules must be followed if readers wish to arrange styles to suit the individual contours of their clients' faces. Study these rules carefully, practise them, and impress on your client that you are confident that you can improve her facial contours by a simple change of hair style. By so doing you are serving two purposes; first, you will gain the confidence of your client, second, by your ability to find a new hair design that suits her, you will increase your patronage through recommendations by well-satisfied clients. A little tact will make your client enthusiastic and interested in your suggestions how a correct hair style will improve her profile.

In these days, showmanship is important, although it must be practised in an appealing manner. Let every one of your patrons know that you are studying *their* particular features; make them "type conscious." But let me repeat that tact is essential in explaining peculiarities of profile, hair line, and shape of head. One cannot say "Madame, you have a pug nose," or "Yours is the type we call a square face." Use a more tactful approach such as "Madame, if you will study your profile, you will notice that you have a very high forehead. I would like to suggest a different hair style that I know will suit you. Let me show you how I propose to dress your hair as I feel certain it will suit you."

Women are always particularly impressed when a hairdresser explains definite fundamental rules for creating the illusion of a good profile, such as harmony of line, balance, etc. A correct approach by you will always give added confidence to your client, who will almost invariably accept your judgment and your ability to design a suitable and artistic hair style for her. To-day more than ever, women like to be fashionable; and with such a variation of artistic hair styles even the most conservative woman can be persuaded to change her hair fashion.

This chapter I consider to be very important, as it provides infinite scope for the imagination and can help an ordinary hairdresser to become a skilled artist. Because hairdressing is an art, it should express in concrete form the correct perspective of the hair, with the face and figure, and emphasise the personality of the individual.

Not all women have perfect features, but the artist must create a style which will emphasise the good characteristics of the face, and camouflage those that are less attractive. A hairdresser should strive for perfection in his work. It must satisfy himself, and thereby achieve the personification of ideal hairdressing. If he can create a style more suitable than that to which his client has been accustomed, and has pleased her, then he has succeeded. "Nothing succeeds like success, competence is established." These are not my words but the expression of a great philosopher.

We know how difficult it is to express certain peculiarities to the individual: some have long thin necks or short stubby ones, some sloping shoulders or protruding ears; all these defects must be given the illusion of being minimized and improved.

The psychological approach to the client is important, and should establish confidence. Analogies may be made. You might say, for example, that you were amazed to see at the theatre the number of inartistic styles, caused mainly by the hairdressers not having studied the individual characteristics. This, in your opinion, could easily have been avoided if the hairdresser had possessed some knowledge of the fundamental principles of physiognomy. After this kind of approach the client will probably be in a receptive mood, and generally willing and enthusiastic to try any style which the hairdresser may suggest to improve her appearance.

The Physiognomy Chart

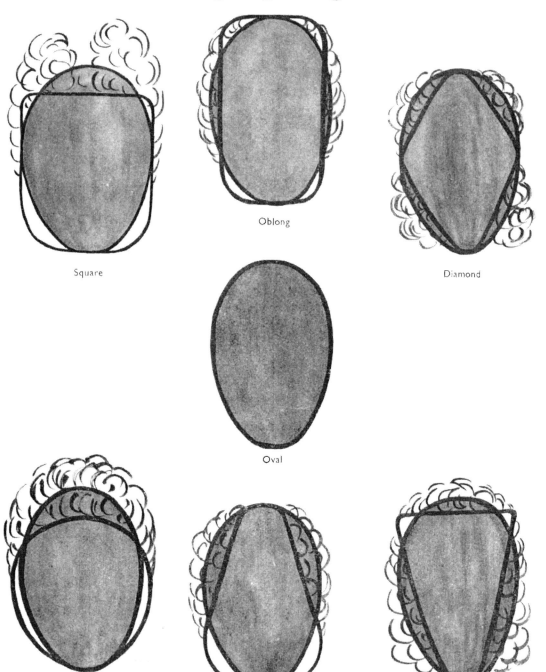

Square

Oblong

Diamond

Oval

Round

Triangle

Inverted Triangle

CHAPTER FOURTEEN

Styling to Type

T HE pendulum of hair fashion is swinging towards the more elaborate styles, and wise women realise this. The creative hairdresser to-day can choose from a wide selection of simple and extravagant designs those which he wishes to display, adding his own variations. A creative hairdresser should design a style in advance of the times and endeavour to predict forthcoming fashions.

One can experiment with hundreds of different interpretations in hairdressing to create a new mode, but good, simple basic styling should be the foundation. Every woman has her own peculiar facial characteristics, and the first consideration for obtaining a suitable style for the individual should be to minimise bad features by drawing attention away from them, and directing it towards the good ones. This, of course, can be done by clever arrangement of the hair, and by comparing the features with the chart illustrated. A careful study of this facial chart will help you to decide in which particular category the contour of a face belongs, thereby enabling you to vary a style so as to focus the attention on those features which should be emphasised. Sometimes the variation is great, sometimes small, but to vary the style successfully, the three fundamentals—practicability, suitability and fashion must predominate.

The accompanying sketches are examples of correct and incorrect styles for different-shaped faces, and are therefore guides on which to base variations of design. The hairdresser must acquire a sufficient sense of artistic ability to enable him to adapt suitable fashions to particular types of features. You must know the reason for your actions, which will be all the better if your capabilities are enhanced and given wider latitude. Analysis and adaptation of the sketches illustrating the "wrong "and "right" coiffure positions for every kind of face, will help you to become a skilled hair-designer. The fortunate woman who is blessed with an oval face can wear any fashionable style with ease and flattery, for the perfect oval is considered the ideal shape for hairdressing.

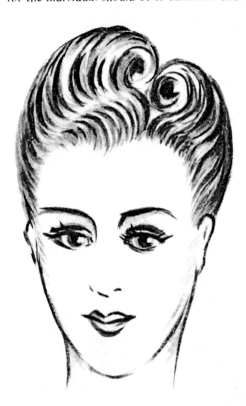

Fig. 72. **Oval.**

66

STYLING TO TYPE

In no other country is more attention paid to the hair than in Great Britain; and unlike other nations there is no set fashion or uniformity in dressing it. Every woman uses her own good taste, and taxes her ingenuity in displaying her hair to the best advantage according to the contour of her face. It is said, "let the oval where it exists be always preserved; where it does not, let the hair be so humoured that the deficiency shall not be perceived."

Although many liberties can be taken in dressing hair for an oval face, there is a limit to the freedom of ideas, and an oval contour can be distorted by an inappropriate style. Practical experience has taught me that placing the hair over the cheeks of an oval face breaks the perfectly-balanced oval line. A centre parting accentuates the beautiful shape.

It is difficult for an inexperienced hairdresser to grasp the importance of this subject at once, but a careful study of the seven sketches will be helpful. They reveal very plainly the alterations in contour that may be achieved by different arrangements of the hair, which should be adjusted to make the face look as oval as possible. You must place the hair where it is needed, and withdraw it where it is not. Each of the types shown in the series of sketches is represented among your clients. Strive to achieve the illusion of the perfect oval by applying the principles outlined. The sketches shown in the following pages have duplicate facial contours, both for the "right" and "wrong" coiffures. You will see that the changes in the facial shapes have been accomplished by the variation of hair styles. I know through my own experience of teaching that students can imbibe this important knowledge quite easily, thereby increasing their confidence and ability.

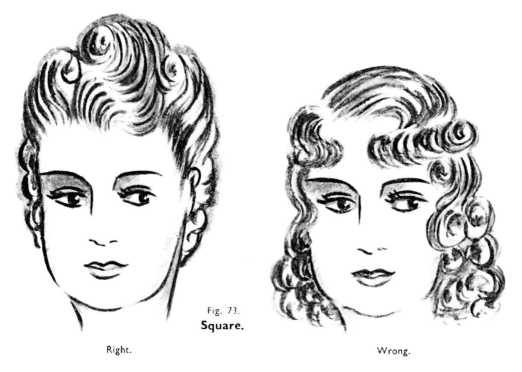

Fig. 73.
Square.

Right.   Wrong.

67

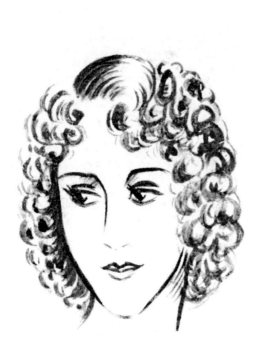

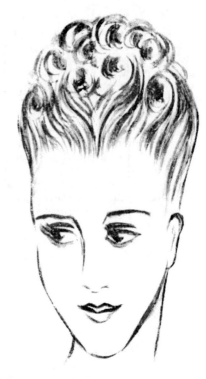

Right.   Fig. 74. **Oblong.**   Wrong.

The Ideal Oval Face. Fig. 72.

The style shown here is smooth, upswept, extremely feminine and flattering, showing the entire shape of the face. It is dignified enough to be worn on any occasion, for day or evening wear, and can be varied in a number of ways, if the natural oval is not distorted. I have chosen the oval face first, because it comes closest to perfection and offers few problems to the stylist.

Formation of pli. Front:—Basic No. 1.
Sides:—Basic No. 3 and 10.

The Square Face. Fig. 73.

This shape is quite common among clients. The top should not be kept flat, and, most important of all, waves must not be formed in a horizontal line, which would have a tendency to make the face more square. A diagonal wave will relieve the square effect. The theory of balanced lines is clearly illustrated in the example shown, by the heightening of the hair to create an illusion of length and thus counteracting the squareness of the features.

Formation of pli. Front:—A diagonal wave as in Basic No. 5 with the pli as in No. 1.
Sides:—Basic No. 7 or No. 10.

STYLING TO TYPE

The Oblong Face. Fig. 74.

One of the characteristics of a long, narrow face is usually that of hollow cheeks. The illusion of a shorter and broader face is achieved by keeping the hair flat on top and fluffing it at the sides. Waves placed horizontally will detract from the long vertical line from the top of head to the tip of the chin. To minimise the sharp features that are often part of a long face, the hair at the sides should be dressed in a soft line towards the face.

Formation of pli. Hair combed well back and kept flat, and a wave as for a "cockscomb" to be placed in between horizontal and diagonal position.

Diamond Shape. Fig. 75.

This embodies the characteristics of a narrow forehead, extreme width at the cheekbones and a narrow, pointed chin. The problems of the diamond-shaped face are not encountered in some other facial types. The narrow areas round the forehead and below the ears should be built out to create the illusion of an oval. The most important part of the work is in making the diamond shape seem to be as oval as possible, thereby lessening the width across the cheekbone. As the face is broad across the centre, a narrowing effect should be obtained by covering a portion of the cheeks with hair, the remainder of the hair being left fairly long and fluffy at the sides to detract from the narrowness of the chin. It is essential that the ears should always be covered. The sketch of the diamond shape in Fig. 75 clearly shows where the hair should be placed to create the right effect.

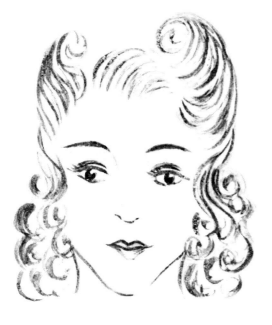
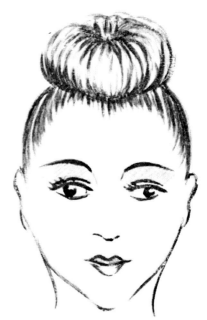

Right. Fig. 75. **Diamond.** Wrong.

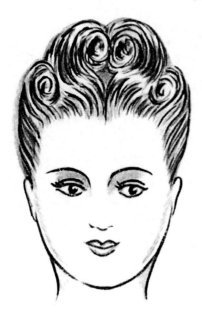

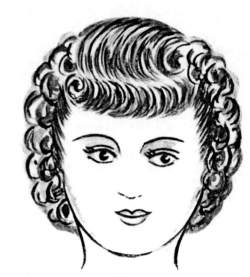

Right.   Fig. 76. **Round.**   Wrong.

The Round Face. Fig. 76.

The fundamental principles for creating a suitable dressing for this type of face are clearly shown in the sketch. You will see the suggestion of an addition of hair to lengthen the contour of the face by piling the hair on top and exposing the ears, thus creating an elongated effect. The design showing a wrong dressing can, of course, be modified to a correct one if an extremely high or raised "bang" is produced. The waved bang must not be placed straight across the forehead but dressed in a round movement with the ends brought upwards towards the head as if for a side-bang. The suggested style as shown has a centre parting with swirls dressed closely together, the object being to create an illusion of length.

The Triangle Shape. Fig. 77.

Characteristics: Narrow forehead, wide jaw and chin line. Object: to create an illusion of width across the forehead and to detract from the jaw line; the dressing should be the the reverse of that given for the inverted triangle. The upper portion of the face must therefore be free from hair or dressed very flat. The suggested style has a fairly flat top, a low wave, with fluffed-out curls which accentuate the width. In this way the broadness of the jaw line is minimised.

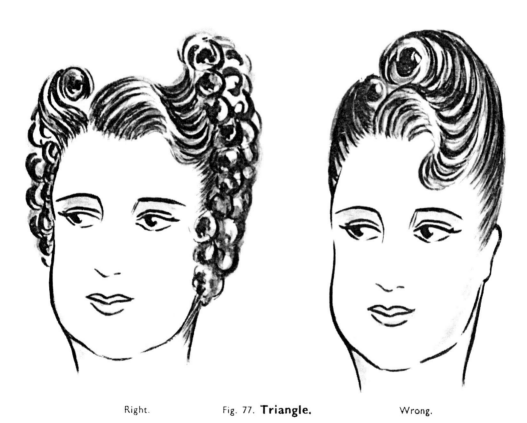

Right.   Fig. 77. **Triangle.**   Wrong.

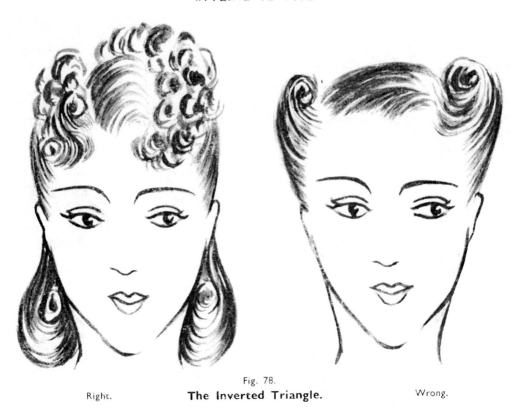

Fig. 78.

Right.   **The Inverted Triangle.**   Wrong.

The Inverted Triangle Shape. Fig. 78.

Characteristics: Narrow chin, wide across the temples. Object: to create an illusion of width on the lower part of the face, and to narrow the head by keeping the hair as flat as possible at the sides. A properly-balanced coiffure for this type of face is essential because most women with a triangular face are very feminine in appearance, due to the small bone formation which makes the chin. Simplicity in the arrangement of the hair style is provided by fluffing the hair low at the sides, thus adding to the width of the lower part of the face. The style suggested in the sketch is a "page-boy" dressing. Alternatively, curls can be easily adapted if a loose design is preferred.

The Normal Head. Fig. 79.

The personality of a woman must be given individuality to achieve a suitable coiffure. She may have a normal shaped head, but may not be able to wear a sophisticated design. To decide the style you must use your judgment.

The desire to be distinctive is always the foremost aim. The sophisticated type of woman with a normal shaped head can wear a dressing more meticulously groomed. On the other hand, the plain woman with a normal shaped head, must have her hair dressed more simply. Profile effect must also be considered to decide the most suitable style so that the height of the dressing as well as the width can be balanced. The theory of balanced lines must always be considered. A short woman cannot wear her hair dressed in the same way as a tall woman, because it may be necessary to dress the former to create a much higher effect.

The style shown on a normal head as the "right" suggestion portrays a well-balanced conception, whereas the "wrong" sketch shows an ungainly shape. This suggested "wrong" design is not condemned because the hair is low on the neck but because the abundance of curls on the front does not balance with the mass of hair at the back—the *tout ensemble* being out of proportion. If the hair had been prepared closely at the back to retain the shape of the head, instead of portraying the severe straightness, and if the curls had been taken off the forehead and placed higher, then a symmetrical arrangement would have been achieved.

After a time all students of hairdressing will study various shapes of heads and consider different features, *i.e.*, protruding ears, shapes of noses, necks (whether they are long and thin, or short and fat), low or high foreheads and other defects in features; these the experienced hair-stylist considers automatically. A coiffure should be as becoming to the back of the head as it is to the face. The dressmaker, for instance, immediately observes her client's disfigurements—the shoulders may be drooping; the neck may be long and thin. The dress-

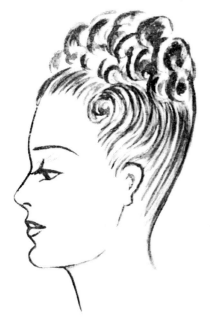

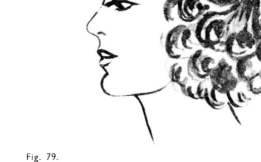

Fig. 79.

Right.   **Normal Head.**   Wrong.

maker designs a dress that will camouflage and improve the figure. The drooping shoulders will be squared with shoulder pads. The long thin neck will appear shorter by clever designing. In the same way, the hairdresser must apply his knowledge and improve the features.

The following illustrations will give you ideas on which to work. Study them carefully; you will notice that facial features as well as the shape of the neck and shoulders play an important part in determining correct hair styles for various types of physiognomy.

Short Thin Neck. Fig. 80.

The object here is to lengthen the neck line by placing the waves diagonally, and to keep the hair high at the nape, thus creating an elongated appearance. If the hair is dressed fluffily at the back and left fairly low, the neckline will not be so noticeable from the back view, but the front effect will, of course, show the shortness from the tip of the ear to the neck line. For this reason I have avoided the long fluffy effect in my illustration.

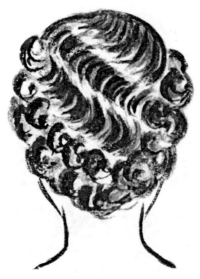
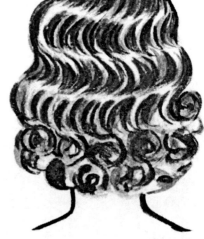

Right.

Fig. 80.

Short Thin Neck.

Wrong.

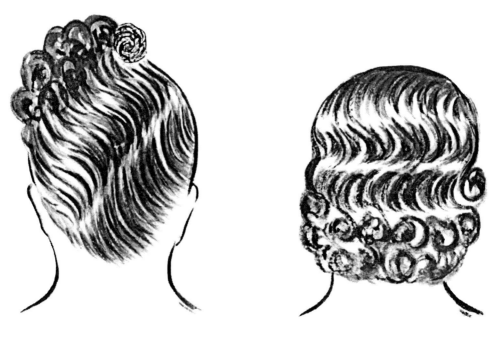

Fig. 81.
Right.   **Short Fat Neck.**   Wrong.

Short Fat Neck. Fig. 81.

Conversely, the important rule to follow for this type is to create an illusion of length to the neck. There is usually a bulge at the nape of the neck, and any hair left low would tend to create width. I do not, therefore, advise curls at the back, for they may seem to be resting on the shoulders, or the bulge may be the only part exposed, and attention will thus be centred entirely on this bad feature. The eye should follow an upward trend, and the waves should preferably be placed in a vertical or diagonal direction. The illustration clearly explains the unattractive shape of the "wrong" design.

Long Thin Neck. Fig. 82.

To achieve correct styling for this type it is essential to minimise the long effect by at least half the length. The unbecoming hollowness which usually accompanies long thin necks should be hidden by placing curls low and trying to cover at least half the neck. The curls must not be dressed in a hard effect; a soft fluffy dressing is desirable. With this type we usually find a narrow head. Therefore your first consideration is to create width and detract from the length. In the previous illustrations you have been shown that vertical waves tend to produce an elongated effect. Therefore to create width, waves placed horizontally will give the illusion of a wider design, and by doing this the ears will be covered. This is important, because a person with a long thin neck has boney spaces behind the ears, which should be completely hidden.

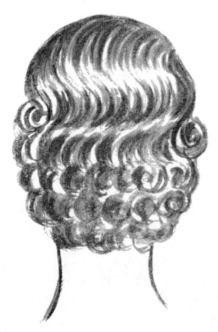 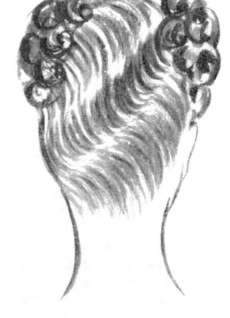

Right.

Fig. 82.

Long Thin Neck.

Wrong.

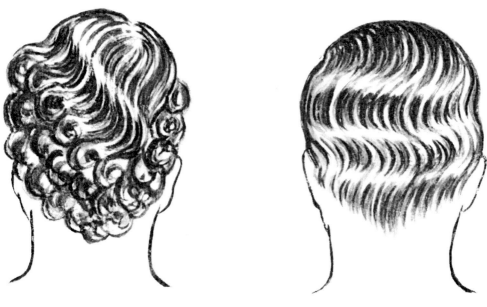

Fig. 83.

Right.　　　**Thick Muscular Neck.**　　　Wrong.

Thick Muscular Neck. Fig. 83.

Experience and practice on various types of irregular features teach us the correct principles to adopt; thus, with a thick muscular neck we must detract from the width. Women with this feature are usually a masculine type, with broad, square shoulders. A hair design should therefore accentuate all the feminine qualities. The style should be practical, and not close to the head because this would make the neck seem to be as wide as the head. As you will observe in the illustration, the short hair design, or an upswept style, would immediately accentuate the short neck. The suggested vertically waved design creates the illusion of a longer and narrower head. The hair should not be waved down horizontally because, as I have said, this design creates width which would be accentuated by the broad shoulders.

STYLING TO TYPE

Creating the Correct Style for Square Shoulders. Fig. 84.

The shape of the shoulders plays an important part in determining the correct hair style. By observing the "wrong" design, you will see that the waves placed horizontally are going in the same direction as the square shoulders. The significance of the shape of the shoulders in relation to the coiffure is important. The general rule must be followed—that any movements having lines parallel to the square shoulders must be avoided, and those having lines at a tangent to the shoulders substituted to detract from the squareness. If the waves are vertical, they will be at right angles to the line of the shoulders. The suggested dressing should be a design, waved and curled in a diagonal movement, which will detract from the squared effect.

The illustration shows an upward dressing, but for the woman who prefers her hair down, the waves must still be placed diagonally. Should curls be desired, then a high cluster of them on the side to which the hair is combed will give the required effect, balanced proportionally.

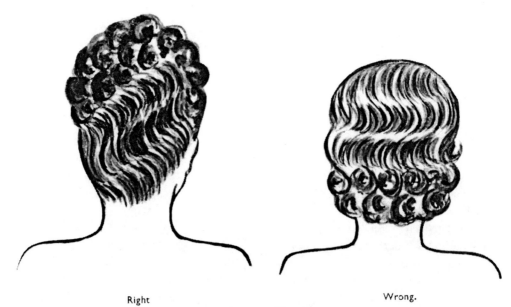

Right   Wrong.

Fig. 84. **Square Shoulders.**

78

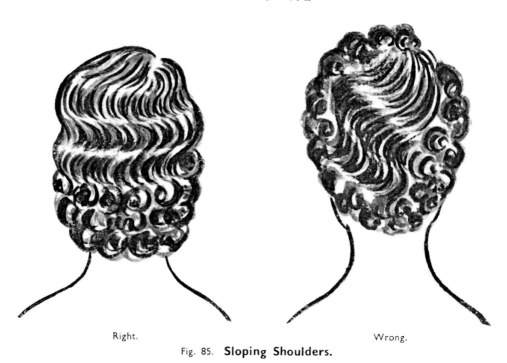

Right.   Wrong.

Fig. 85. **Sloping Shoulders.**

Creating the Correct Style for Sloping Shoulders. Fig. 85.

By analysing drooping or sloping shoulders, you will observe that they tend to make the neck seem unusually long.   To satisfy a client's very natural desire to minimise this defect, you must create or adapt a style which will give the drooping shoulders a square effect. Always try to achieve an improved effect by avoiding any lines that run parallel to the sloping shoulders.   By placing the waves in a horizontal position you will help to give a squared appearance, whereas you will notice that the "wrong" illustration is accentuated still further by the diagonal waves running parallel with the shoulders, thus drawing attention to the sloping effect.   Curls arranged low at the neck will make the head seem to be nearer to the shoulders as the unusually long line of the sloping shoulders, especially with a hair style diagonally waved, gives the appearance of the head being too far from the shoulders.   This should be avoided.

STYLING TO TYPE

Low Forehead.   Fig. 86.

The lowness of the forehead should not be revealed.   It is a common error to comb the hair right up giving it a sleek effect.   An abundance of curls over the hair line at the front and at the nape of the neck provides the right effect.   To prove that a coiffure can be marred if it is not scientifically carried out, notice a client who has a low forehead.   She will not be happy if you give her a style that shows the narrowness in its entirety.

From the variation of modern styles choose one which will hide all the bad points and show to full advantage the good ones.   When the hair is placed in accordance with the features you improve the *tout ensemble*.   In my "right" illustration I have suggested the placing of a high "bang" that just covers the forehead hair line.   The hair at the back could be taken down, but avoid any fullness on the face.   In the "wrong" dressing you will notice that the hair line is fully exposed, the wave is heavy, and the "page-boy" is too far on the face.   I am not condemning the "page-boy" dressing because of the low forehead, but this could be modified to be practical if the dressing of the "page-boy" was taken back exposing the ears a little, and the front dressed higher as suggested with a high "bang" or a cluster of curls.   The object of taking the hair back to expose the ears is to lengthen the small jaw line which usually accompanies a narrow forehead.

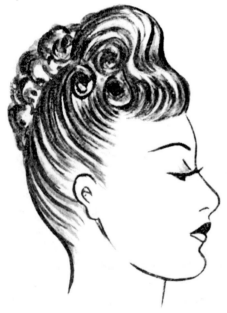

Fig. 86.
Low Forehead.

Right   Wrong.

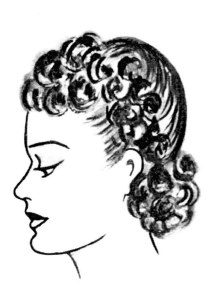

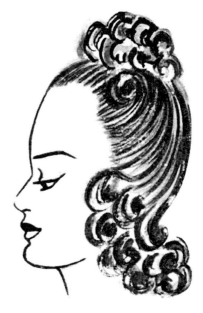

Right.

Fig. 87.
**High Forehead.
Short Chin.**

Wrong.

High Forehead with Short Chin. Fig. 87.

It does not necessarily follow that a woman with a high forehead must also have a small or short chin. Practical experience of hair designing to type has already taught us that a high forehead can be given a smaller effect by lowering the dressing on to the forehead. When a short chin is pronounced and is accompanied by a high forehead, the long vertical line from forehead to the chin must be broken by lowering the hair line to shorten the length from the front hair to the chin. By placing waves in a horizontal position you break the long vertical line. If the ears are exposed, this alone will lengthen the short jaw line.

STYLING TO TYPE

Turned-up Nose, Straight Profile.   Fig. 88.

The discriminating hairdresser who wishes to create a gracefully-proportioned design to suit his client's features finds the defects of this profile difficult to counteract.   It is easier to attempt an elaborate arrangement of a hair style which may be lovely for evening wear, but more difficult to design a practical dressing for everyday wear.   As the profile is straight and flat, the waves should be dressed high, pointing towards the nose, so that it is given an illusion of length.   To widen the facial area, the hair should be taken off the face, and the ears exposed.   Horizontal waves should not be introduced as this would give the square-headed effect shown in the "wrong" sketch.

Hook Nose and Receding Brow.   Fig. 89.

The fortunate women whose features are regular can wear any style with ease, but those with a hook nose and receding brow need an effective camouflage to improve the imperfect features.   To decide on the most becoming position of the hair for this type, care must be taken against lengthening still further the line from the tip of the hook nose to the hair line of the receding brow.   This should be your first consideration.   With this type it is a common mistake to place waves in the same direction as the hook of the nose.   Attention must be detracted from the nose by minimising its length.   A psychological problem may be created by the client's knowledge that her type makes it difficult for her to wear elaborate modern creations.

This psychological problem can be overcome by the hairdresser if he shows her that these styles need not be unbecoming if they are balanced by basic movements which incorporate the fundamental principles of styling to type to suit her face.

Throughout this book you will notice that I am constantly emphasising the importance of studying a woman's personality and individuality.   This study is important with every facial type, but more particularly so with women who have a hook nose and receding brow. They are usually of the sophisticated type and are liable to exaggerate their hair styles.   The "wrong" illustration clearly shows this exaggeration.   By creating a suitable, appropriate style, the hook nose and the receding chin can be considerably minimised as the illustration shows.

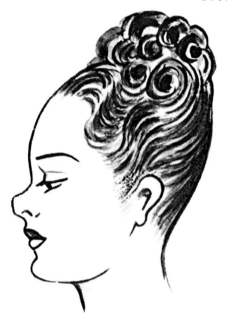

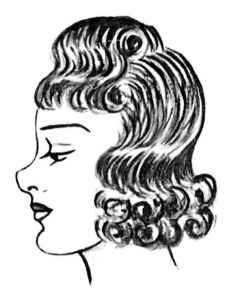

Fig. 88.

Right.   **Turned-up Nose, Straight Profile.**   Wrong.

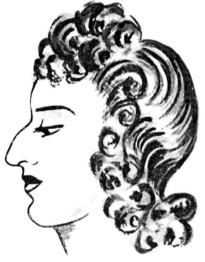

Fig. 89.

Right.   **Hook Nose, Receding Brow.**   Wrong.

STYLING TO TYPE

Receding Brow and Chin. Fig. 90.

The rule of physiognomy to minimise bad features by drawing attention away from them, will prove to be an important factor when dressing the hair of a person of the type shown in this sketch. Your client knows full well that certain styles are impossible to wear, and cannot therefore follow fashionable modes. Most probably you have never taken much notice of the real difficulty that arises with a person with such features, but now I hope that the subject of "Styling to Type" has stimulated your artistic feelings, and by a careful perusal of contour expression you will know at a glance that for this type, waves or movements should never be on a line with the nose. Observe carefully the illustration; you will notice that the nose projects prominently forward, overbalancing the chin. Therefore to shorten the line from the tip of the nose to the back of the head, the waves should follow a downward curve, with the hair brought forward to the face. The ears should be covered to shorten the long line from the tip of the nose to the ear in the same way as by placing curls at the nape there is a tendency to make the appearance of a longer movement from the tip of the chin to the back of the head. The receding brow can be minimised by bringing the hair forward, either a high bang or soft curls well down on the forehead.

Square Jaw and Small Nose. Fig. 91.

Women with these characteristics are almost invariably of the masculine type, and every possible effort should be made to produce a feminine appearance. With this type you will usually find a wide forehead. The object here is to cover the ears and soften the jaw-line. To give the small nose a longer appearance, a wave should be placed on the forehead, as for a "cockscomb," and should be in a diagonal line. This diagonal line of the wave will counteract the square line of the jaw, and, if placed just above the eye, will make the forehead seem narrower.

Simplicity of line is of primary importance when carrying out designs of distinction. The rules must be governed by fashion changes. These frequently start by one artistic creation meeting the approval of other women who demand a similar style from their own hairdresser. Styles of hairdressing are as much the concern of the public as of the trade. If the public demand a variety of artistic creations the trade must supply them. The basic principle for styling to type is undoubtedly a good foundation for learning the study of the higher technical science of hairdressing. It is an essential step towards acquiring that expert knowledge for which every hairdresser aims. It is only in this way that confidence can be gained. Once it is gained, the power of handling new ideas will ensure the cultivation and retention of a more exclusive clientele.

I have not covered all the points of styling for irregular features. Much more could be said on this subject for there are of course other facial differences for which variations in hair styling are necessary.

Remember always that because a client has intuition, foresight and ideas of her own, her co-operation is often most helpful in creating a suitable style.

84

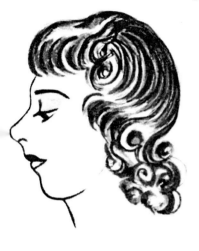

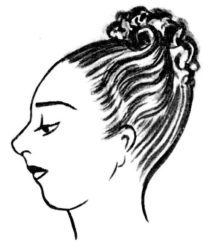

Fig. 90.

Right.   **Receding Brow and Chin.**   Wrong.

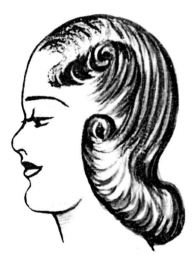

Fig. 91.

Right.   **Square Jaw and Small Nose.**   Wrong.

CHAPTER FIFTEEN

Adapting Postiche to Modern Hairdressing

SCARCELY any study of social conditions in history is more expressive than a survey of hairdressing fashions. This is a vast subject and could not be covered in one lesson; each country and every generation could scarcely be described adequately in one lecture.

The present-day mode of adding false hair is a revival of a custom adopted many years ago. I have seen some old and lovely pictures showing ladies adorned with fascinating curls and plaits. Some very becoming hairdressings and inspirations from Ancient Greece are often incorporated in our present-day fashions.

Among the remarkable Greek hairdressings that have inspired us are those of Diana, Venus, Daphne, Psyche and many others of equally artistic merit.

The English period of 1800 was especially interesting because the hair was worn short, similar to that of to-day, with false curls which were arranged differently from the present fashion.

The year 1830 became a landmark in the history of hairdressing. The famous loop dressing, plaits interlaced with curls, was introduced by Croisat.

To-day, women are wearing postiche to complete an up-to-date stylish mode. The addition of false hair can make a lady's head dignified and becoming if, of course, it is placed artistically and in the correct position. The principle in the arrangement of hair around the forehead should be to preserve or assist the oval form of face. As this differs with different individuals the treatment should be adapted accordingly if the balance and symmetry of the outline are not to be marred.

To be fashionable is always a personal necessity, but in the quest of fashion nothing really new is created as all styles are a repetition of history. The art of wigmaking goes back many years. The making of ringlets, braids, curls and plaits is a specialised art, and the manufacturers can make any design to the colour required.

I have included a few designs of styling with plaits which I think you will find interesting. Many variations can be carried out. Switches or tails of hair can be of the two, three or four stem variety. The two stem can be used for making a figure 8 at the nape, or a cross-over coil. The three or four plaited switch is the most popular one for the present-day fashion. A bunch or cluster of curls makes an interesting variation. Many of the glamorous coiffures seen on the films are achieved by the clever use of extra pieces of hair. They are dressed to supply any additional part of a hair style, to produce length or height or a quick change from one style to another.

At present there is a growing trend for women to wear postiche; this addition gives a more elegant look to a head and also transforms a day dressing into an elaborate evening style. All you require to solve the problems of applying postiche is a selection of hair pieces and a knowledge of how to apply them.

The knowledge derived from manipulating postiche will provide excellent education and instruction. The art of plaiting the hair is not difficult once the principles of movements are

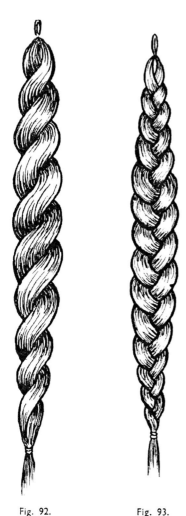

Fig. 92.

Two stem switch, coiled and crossed over.

Fig. 93.

Three stem switch, plaited.

mastered. There is no end to the variety of charming designs that may be accomplished. The following diagrams will help you. It is advisable to practise the various forms of plaiting on thick pieces of string if switches of hair are not available.

Two Stem Switch. Fig. 92.

A very attractive design known as the "Cable Coil," "Hollow Twist" or "Coiled Coronet" can easily be done with the two stem switch. This is accomplished in the following manner. To thicken the stem of hair, back-comb it and brush lightly making sure the hair is smooth.

The object of making a hollow twist is to create a larger and circular coil. Place the hair in the left hand, and the first finger of the right hand as close to the top of the switch as possible. Give a light twist over the first finger allowing the hair to fall over it. Place the fingers of the left hand underneath the forefinger of the right hand, remove this finger and replace with the left hand fingers. The right hand thumb is then placed in the coil with the fingers on the top of the hair. Turn the right hand in a semi-circle and gently remove the left hand. Place the left hand under the right hand, putting the fingers in line with the right thumb and then throw the hair over the fingers of the left hand and replace the right thumb as before in the hollow coil. Repeat each movement in the same manner, using the left fingers to obtain the correct hollowness as the twist proceeds.

Should the hair be well tapered, fluff or back-comb the ends more before making the hollow twist, to give the ends a fuller effect. It is advisable, when making a figure 8, to pin securely the first coil made by forming a loop, the end going towards the centre. When both loops are made, the ends are tucked underneath.

For a cross-over hollow twist, take the ends of the coil in each hand, the left hand holding the ends of the coil between the first and second

87

fingers, and the right hand holding the hair between the thumb and first finger. Cross the hair from the right over the left in a twisting movement, catching the right coil under the left thumb, the left coil being held now in the right hand. Repeat the previous instruction of holding the ends, and complete to the end of the coil. To secure the ends together, twist cotton round or back-comb the ends together.

Three Stem Plait. Fig. 93.

The hair should be well brushed and combed before you begin to plait. To thicken each stem, back-comb and brush smoothly. Hold the left and right strand in their respective hands, place the centre strand between first and second fingers of the left hand. Then place the right strand in the centre over the first finger. The right hand will now be holding the centre strand. Place the left strand into the centre, repeating the above procedure. The ends are securely tied or back-combed.

Four Stem Plait. Figs. 94 and 95.

Always take the stem at the extreme right, pass over one, under one, over one—continuing this order to the end. Plait as tightly or as loosely as the design requires. Constant practice is essential.

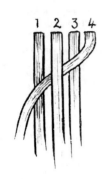

Fig. 94.
Making a Four Stem Plait

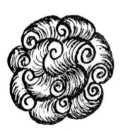

Fig. 96.
Cluster of curls knotted
on circular net

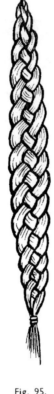

Fig. 95.
Four stem switch
plaited

Adapting Curls for Hair Styling. Fig. 96.

Various styles can be introduced with the addition of curls. They can be placed on the crown, the front of the head, on one side to give a one-sided dressing, or placed in the nape of the neck. When a lady has had her hair cut and decides to grow it again, the addition of curls on the neck would cover the growing hair. The length of hair most practical for obtaining a cluster of curls or large puff curls should be approximately six inches. The curls should be made either on weft, or knotted on a circular net which should be about two inches wide. The method of curling should be on bigoudis as explained in Fig. 8.

ADAPTING POSTICHE TO MODERN HAIRDRESSING

A Bow as Hair Ornament.

Adding a bow made of ribbon or velvet to a completed dressing has been very popular for the last few years. Women yearn for the occasional glamour that can be achieved by the addition of ornaments. A bow made of ribbon that can be bought at any store does not create the same individuality as that of a bow of human hair. An effective yet becoming simplicity is added to the entire ensemble, as seen on page 148. The bow ornament is simple to make. Three narrow marteaux are necessary—two approximately nine inches long and the other about four inches. Back-comb each marteaux, making a loop of the long ones, and join together by pinning. Then take the short piece of hair and wrap it over the centre. To keep all the ends neat and intact, spray a little lacquer over the bow.

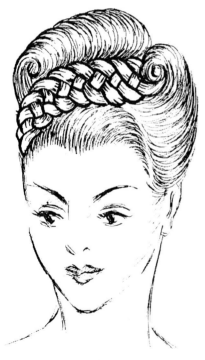

Fig. 97.
Adaption of a Four Stem Plait.

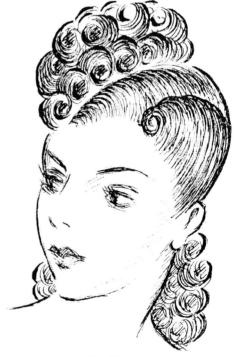

Fig. 98.
A Dressing incorporating False Curls.

CHAPTER SIXTEEN

"*The Cockscomb*"

THE "Cockscomb" coiffure has been most practical for a number of years, but women still consider this style to be very effective and becoming. One of the most important features of this design is the lightness of its appearance. The "Cockscomb" can be adapted to a number of different designs; it can, in fact, be elaborated to a mode of exceptional artistic expression.

This design would be futile to women with low foreheads—it would make a forehead look too heavy. The woman with a high forehead can wear a "Cockscomb," as it will make her forehead seem narrower. A woman with a wide face could wear this style with simplicity, as it would remove a certain amount of heaviness that would otherwise fall on the temples.

One of the fundamentals of this dressing is the correct way of cutting the amount of

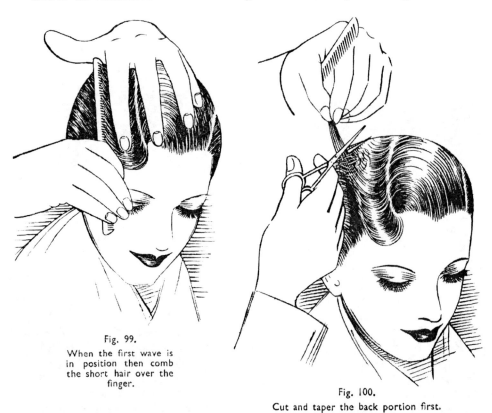

Fig. 99.
When the first wave is in position then comb the short hair over the finger.

Fig. 100.
Cut and taper the back portion first.

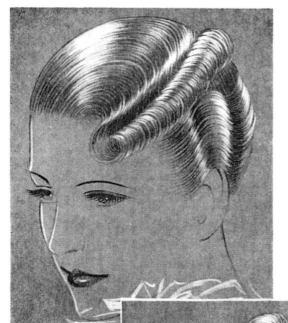

hair necessary for the "Cockscomb." The most practical design is the one illustrated in Fig. 99. The rudimentary principles must be carried out scientifically, or instead of being an artistic coiffure it will be a heavy and unbalanced headdress.

The Setting Instruction for the "Cockscomb."

The hair is combed back off the face revealing the entire hair line. The first wave is placed in position as if for a two dip design. Fig. 99 shows the first wave in position with the rest of the hair combed well back. Keep the forefinger in this position, make a parallel parting with a tail comb and comb the hair for the "Cockscomb"

Fig. 101.
A "Cockscomb" coiffure with the sides waved off the face.

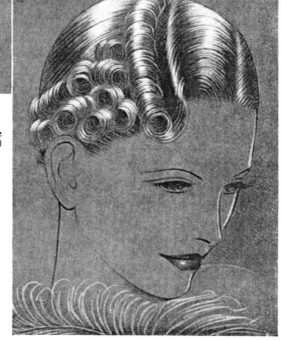

Fig. 102.
A similar design favouring curls at the sides. (Important: note how the hair is taken well back off the forehead in all the "Cockscomb" designs)

91

THE "COCKSCOMB"

Fig. 102 favours curls at the sides; the back portion is kept perfectly straight. This design is very becoming with short hair which can be swathed across the back from the small side, the ends finishing in curls. The dressing shown in Fig. 101 is practical, and will meet the demands of discriminating women.

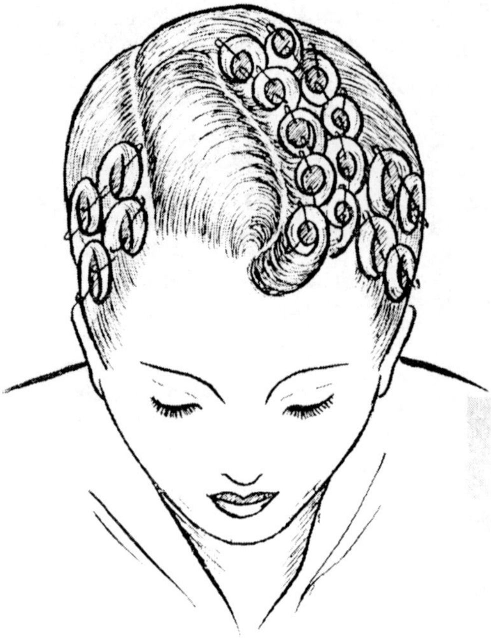

Fig. 103.

over this finger. Having previously prepared the hair to the correct length desired for the "Cockscomb," it will readily respond to the combing over the finger. Should there not be any short hair, or supposing it necessitates a first time cutting for this design, then the method of procedure is the one shown in Fig. 100. As you will observe, the wave is placed in position: ascertain the length of "Cockscomb" required, then cut and taper, beginning at the end of the "Cockscomb," as shown in the illustration. When the hair is thoroughly dry, comb through and roll over finger. The finished coiffure is shown in Figs. 101 and 102. A great variation of different designs can be introduced with a "Cockscomb," and this should prove conclusively that unique effects can be achieved by differentiating existing modes through the addition of waves and curls as in figs. 103 and 104.

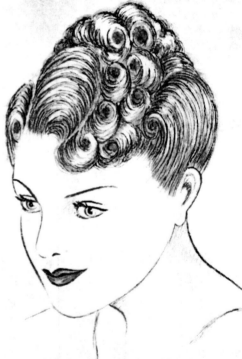

Fig 104. Showing a "Cockscomb" movement, curls high on crown, large sweep at sides.

CHAPTER SEVENTEEN

Variations of the "Bang"

THE basic principle of a good design lies
in the correct formation of the pli.
The "Bang" is an excellent example of
making waves by the pin-curl method, and
with the help of these sketches readers
should be able to achieve, without difficulty,
the various designs of the "Bang," which
are so popular to-day.

The correct placing of the curls allows
you to guide a wave in the direction you
wish it to follow in the finished movement.
The size of the wave depends on the curli-
ness of the hair and the size of the curl
made. Hair that has been permanently

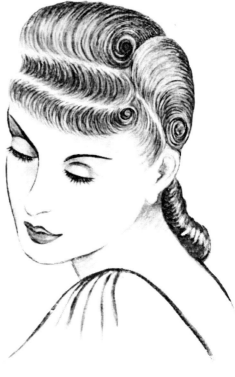

Fig. 106.

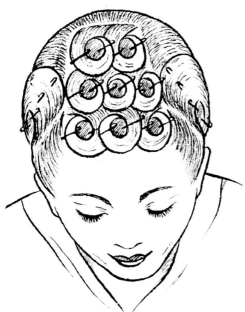

Fig. 105. First row combed down, two C curls and
one CC. The remaining curls are CC curls.
Sides. Basic No. 8.

waved, or very naturally curly hair, should
be made into larger curls; otherwise a frizzy
or small wave will result. Well-made curls
will always ensure well-made waves.

The length of hair most suitable for a
"Bang" should be approximately six to
eight inches, with the ends well-tapered.
The principles illustrated here show the
correct way to pin the curls, so that when
combed out they form a neatly waved
"Bang." A careful study of the four

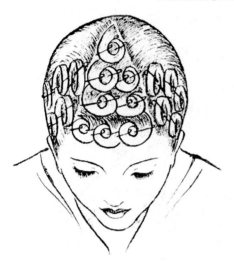

Fig. 107. "Bang" for high forehead. *Sides.* Basic No. 10.

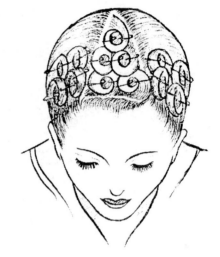

Fig. 108. "Bang" for low forehead. *Sides.* Basic No. 10.

variations I have submitted will teach you how to place the curls according to the width of the forehead.

Fig. 106 shows a high effect from the crown, and by reverse curling a tighter wave is produced. Divide the hair evenly on both sides, narrowing the division towards the crown. Part the hair in even sections for three rows of curls. The first row is combed down and placed in clockwise curls over the hair line. The number of curls must be determined by the amount of curl in the hair and the size of wave required. As you will see in the pli of Fig. 105, two curls in the front are in a *C* movement, and the third curl in a *CC* position. This third curl is so placed in this position to simplify the dressing out. The remaining two rows are placed in *CC* curls brought down towards the face.

Fig. 109 is similar to Fig. 106. The hair is divided to form a triangle. These two illustrations, Fig. 107 and Fig. 108 show variations for a high or low forehead.

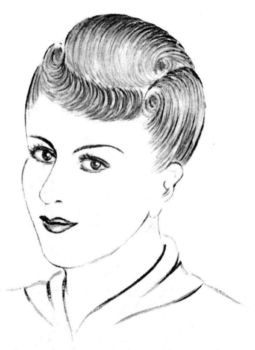

Fig. 109. A high waved "Bang" with long side sweep.

94

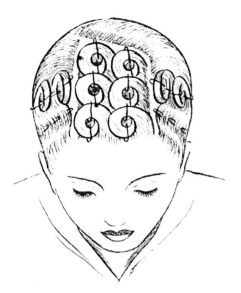

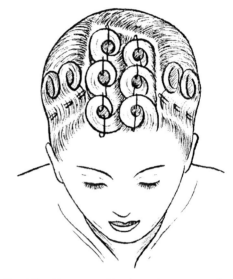

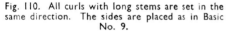

Fig. 110. All curls with long stems are set in the same direction. The sides are placed as in Basic No. 9.

Fig. 111. Reverse curling for a deeper wave is shown. The sides are as in Basic No. 9.

The crest of the wave in Fig. 108 will help considerably in the dressing out as it will keep the hair more upright from the head, and there will be less tendency to drop low over the forehead should the hair be rather long.

Fig. 112 is known as the "side bang" as the wave is dressed out to the side. This very popular style lends itself to various artistic designs. The two different pli formations should be carefully studied. The layout of the front curls in Fig. 110 will produce a much larger waved movement than the reverse curling in Fig. 111. Both plis are dressed out in the same way. Both methods should be practised to satisfy the requirements of your individual clients. Waves are important. They are flattering to the face and they are pliable, so that you can create many variations from one basic foundation.

Fig. 113 shows a "bolster" or "rolled bang." In the previous variations under this heading the front effect is done first, but the dressing for the front for the "bolster" is done last. The tape is placed round the head, holding the front hair in position, while the ends are rolled *under* on a crepe hair bigoudi. The ends of the bigoudi are brought round as in Fig. 114. The length of the section is determined by the thickness of the rolled bang. This section can be placed into waves before the tape is tied.

Another way of creating the "bolster bang" is shown in Fig. 115. Complete the back and sides before placing the tape. It is important to comb the hair from the sides of the section towards the centre before tying the tape. This applies to Fig. 114 and Fig. 115. The pli for Fig. 115 presents standing up curls in the front with one curl on each side. This separate curl will help the roundness of the "rolled bang."

95

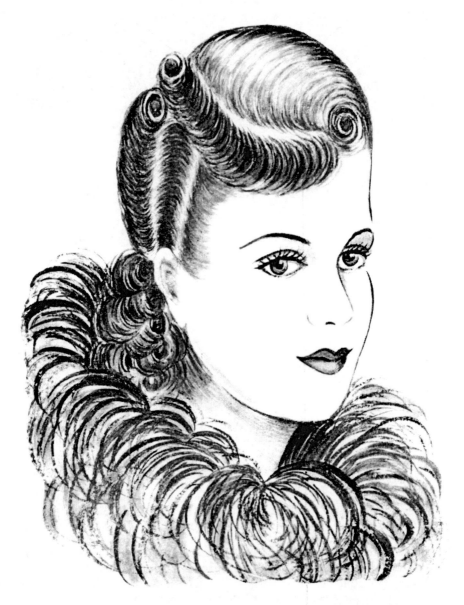

Fig. 112. The completed "Side Bang" Movement with Basic No. 9 at sides.

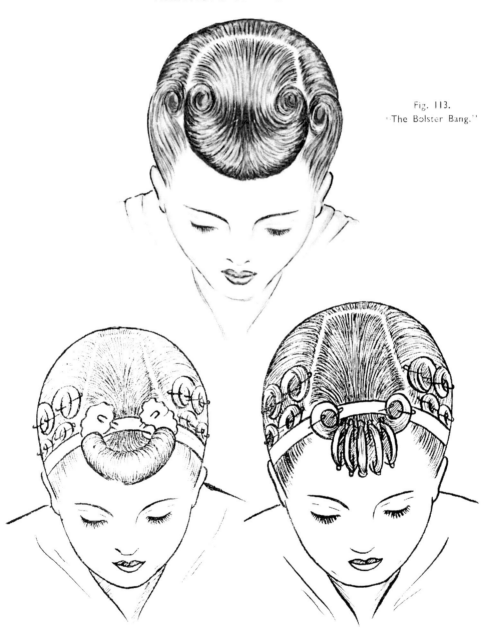

Fig. 113.
"The Bolster Bang."

Fig. 114. The sides and back are completed before tape is tied. Shape the hair first before rolling bigoudi.

Fig. 115. The pli is prepared as in Fig. 114, standing up curls in front, rolled under.

97

VARIATIONS OF THE "BANG"

Dressing out the "Bang"

COMBING and dressing-out a carefully-planned design gives the hairdresser distinct pleasure. But I have frequently noticed that many hairdressers are nervous and cautious when combing out a pin-curl setting. Since the final dressing is so important, and affects the result of the coiffure, it cannot be given too much attention. Correct dressing should not necessarily take a great deal of time. The more you learn about the technique of final dressing, the more time you will save.

Nevertheless, good combing results cannot, of course, be achieved unless the pli has been correctly executed. Back-combing is recommended for most present-day styling as it enables the hairdresser to mould into shape the planned conception. The design in Fig. 106 shows a high effect which can be achieved only by back-combing at the roots. A flat dressing would not be satisfactory to the wearer as it would then fall too low over the forehead. To ensure smooth styling, comb and brush the section for the "Bang." With the tail comb make a division across the head near the crown, lift high and back-comb down to the scalp. Treat the remaining section in a similar manner, dividing the hair and back-combing well at the roots.

Should the hair be very thick, about four sections for back-combing would be necessary. It is important to back-comb each strip of hair backwards, away from the face; this will ensure the height required. When each section has been back-combed thoroughly at the roots and lightly to the ends, a brush should be swept backwards over the whole to achieve smoothness *under* the "Bang" as well as on the surface. Now the hair is held all together and brought forward over the left hand towards the face, brushed lightly to ensure the surface hair is really smooth, and then given a final back-comb underneath close to the head.

The left hand is now placed high or low on the brow (depending upon the position of the "Bang" on the forehead) and the whole mesh of hair is combed over it. The back of the left hand should be kept close to the face so that the ridge of the first wave can be moulded over the palm with the comb, which is held in the right hand. Keep the teeth of the comb under this ridge to control the hair, slip the left hand gently away, and press with the fingers under the first ridge on to the brow. Form another crest with the comb and slide the fingers of the left hand down to hold it in position. Finally, feather-out the finished edge of the last wave with the comb and complete the dressing with a decorative curl on the brow. Should the hair be rather long, then tuck the ends under the last wave.

CHAPTER EIGHTEEN

The "Side Swirl"

E VERY student must achieve proficiency in curl manipulation. Nothing is really appreciated until you have reached the highest possible standard. The finest hair stylists continue to practise new conceptions of hair design. Artistic coiffures, whether practical or for evening wear, are based on the curl method; the technical foundation for each style is therefore a complete study on its own. In the "Side Swirl," you will find that the shape and foundation of the curls are the basis of your guidance; the curls will prove both simple and artistic, and many variations can be produced from this pli. You could evolve many designs for the front dressing,

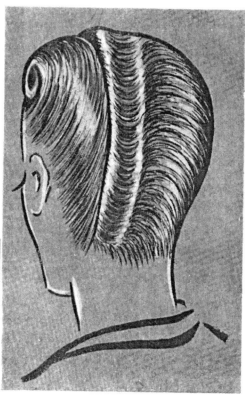

Fig. 116. The "Side Swirl" is overlapping the curls made near the crest.

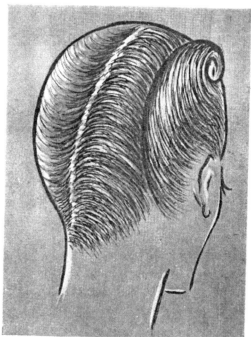

Fig. 117. The "Side Swirl" with swathed vertical waved back.

incorporating the back "Side Swirl." It is advisable to complete the front pli first, and then continue with the back.

Divide off the hair required for the upward sweeps. This parting should extend to the neck, not too far towards the centre. The hair is then combed across to the other side. The first movement is an upward wave, making only one complete wave in a vertical line; place pins in this

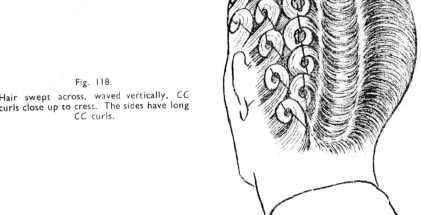

Fig. 118.

Hair swept across, waved vertically. CC curls close up to crest. The sides have long CC curls.

wave to keep it secure while curling. The curls are then placed counter clockwise close to the crest. The sides are then completed in swirl curls, fairly long *CC* stems on the left side, and long *C* curls on the right side.

The Dressing Out

Complete your front design. Comb the back hair across, also comb out the curls. As this design calls for a high movement it is essential to do extra back-combing at the roots. Make diagonal partings, back-comb, gradually lift the hair whilst doing so. Brush into position, so that the sweep lies close to the head. You will find that while placing the hair into position, the curls which were placed near the wave get interlocked when the side sweep is combed into position.

CHAPTER NINETEEN

The Side-Swept "V" Roll

Technical education is not now available in London at hairdressing academies as it was when there were numerous societies and teaching organisations. There were many opportunities to learn and gain technical information from the experienced stylists, for the progressive hairdresser is always anxious to learn how to execute hair styles, whether practical or the more elaborate designs.

Various essential points must be taken into consideration, such as the fundamental rules of varying the abundance of hair where the hair is flat, or flattening the hair at positions where the hair is inclined to be full. A great number of women favour off the face styles, also the hair up at the back, or the tendency slightly to brush up off the hair line; but fashion does not alter the fact that line of shape is the first consideration.

The dressing included here shows an example of hair design in accordance with its title, the Side Swept "V" Roll. Readers should not copy this design without first of all ascertaining whether it will suit the lady. This hair style is a perfect example of following rules of shape for a complete *ensemble*, is one of effective simplicity, and is admirably suitable for both young and middle-aged.

Setting Instructions.

The frontal effect is not shown in this illustration. Readers will either have to introduce a design from the numerous suggestions in this publication or use their own ideas. It is advisable to complete the front pli first of all. Make a division, as shown, to the centre of the nape of the neck as shown in Fig. 120. Brush the hair across, begin with an upward wave, and make a vertical wave slightly on a slant. C curls are then made closely to the crest as shown in Fig. 121. Divide the hair on the left side and place into position CC curls with fairly long stems overlapping the divisional parting. The hair left on the right side is also placed into position with long stems into C curls slightly overlapping the curls already done. The frontal sides can be designed as in Basic No. 10.

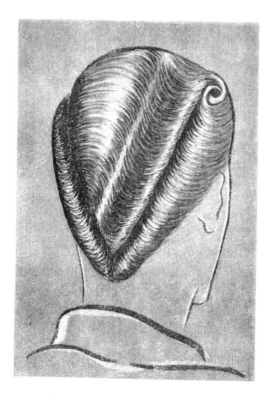

Fig. 119. The Side-Swept "V" Roll.

The Dressing Out

There is a great art in the dressing out of any hair style, but in this particular design especially, great importance must be attached to the dressing out. Complete your frontal design. Comb the hair as set, across the side, and comb out loosely all the curls. Should a larger "V" roll be required, then the hair must be back-combed. You can vary the sides in the front, either by a separate swirl or individual swirled curls, or comb into position to form a roll down to the nape, making an elongated roll. Place the first finger on the head, extending level with the crest of the wave, the right hand combing upwards over the first finger. The waved side is always easier to roll over as the swirl curls overlap the

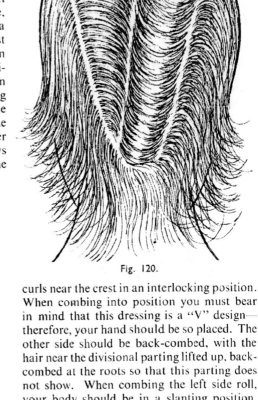

Fig. 120.

curls near the crest in an interlocking position. When combing into position you must bear in mind that this dressing is a "V" design— therefore, your hand should be so placed. The other side should be back-combed, with the hair near the divisional parting lifted up, back-combed at the roots so that this parting does not show. When combing the left side roll, your body should be in a slanting position, your fingers pointing to the centre of the nape. As with the other side, the hair is rolled and tucked in over the first finger. Make sure the ends meet to a point at the centre of the nape. A very neat design on this principle may be achieved without the wave, the hair being swept straight across. The preparation for the pli is similar in operation, by making a slight crest for the position of *C* curls. The hair for this style is therefore combed downwards from the left side division.

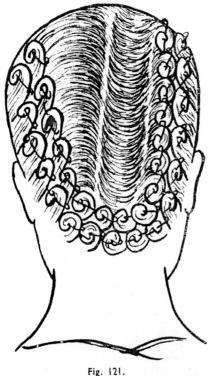

Fig. 121.

CHAPTER TWENTY

The "Page Boy"

ALTHOUGH there is no recognised standard of efficiency or technique in hairdressing, certain definite rules must be adhered to. The most important rule is shape, without which all the artistic manipulations and conceptions are futile.

The "Page Boy" design illustrated here, is a simple and dignified coiffure. Despite the continued popularity of this design, a great number of hairdressers have not given it a welcome They maintain that the turned-under effect is unprofitable, because of its easy manipulation for the client. As I see it, however, there is, and always will be, a welcome for new ideas; whether a design is a "Page Boy" or an "Edwardian," it should be known by all.

The "Page Boy" is considered to be an easy style. Radical changes in hair styles have been few and far between these last few years, but if the "Page Boy" suits the wearer it can express originality. Hairdressers and clients often adopt the "Page Boy" regardless of type and suitability. This, of course, is against all the principles of correctness and smartness. The "Page Boy" coiffure can be worn for day and evening wear, and can be arranged with great chic, thus giving your client a suggestion of a new design, easy to manipulate and distinctive.

Because this dressing has a tendency to suggest length, it should not be used on a woman with a long face; the long, sloping back and under-curl would accentuate the length.

The length of hair for the "Page Boy" design is an important factor in the creation of the right shape. In this style, short hair gives the appearance of squareness at the back, whereas the object is to lengthen the shape.

There are many variations of designs, and the examples of the following sketches are suggestions for movement and pattern which will cover most creations on the line of the "Page Boy" design. Great care should be taken in the tapering for this style. The full length of the hair at the back must be maintained, but the underneath hair can be tapered so that the roll-under movement will be more effective and easier to manipulate.

"Page Boy" Setting Instructions

The Step-by-Step development for this design will be clearly understood by following the sketches. Fig. 122 has been prepared and combed ready for setting. It is as well to mention here that the hair has been cut and tapered to the correct shape. Observe the shortness at the sides gradually getting longer in a round movement as you approach the bottom of the back hair. Comb the hair from the crown straight down, shape the sides in a semi-circular movement. This shaping is most important because it is the preliminary to most "Page Boy" designs to obtain a more beautiful effect.

It is advisable in most cases to complete the frontal design before doing the back. As an example therefore of a front movement not shown elsewhere in the book, Fig. 126 is a simple design with two large *CC* curls and one *C* curl on the small side. The number of curls can, of course, be varied according to the thickness of the hair. When the front is completed then the side movement, which is Basic No. 8, is placed in position. Continue with the back, beginning with the top curls as in Fig. 123, and carry on down to the sides as shown. Place a tape at the nape, over the ears and tied in the front, as in Fig. 124; place

103

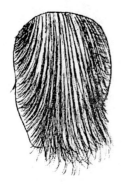

Fig. 122.

Hair combed straight down the sides, shaped towards the front.

a piece of cotton wool under the knot; this will prevent marking the forehead. Place a fairly large curl over the tape on each side of the neck. Do not have the remaining hair very wet—only a slight dampness is sufficient—and roll up on a bigoudi which is a round pad made of crepe hair. The size of the rolled-under effect is determined by the size of the crepe bigoudi used. The shorter the hair the thinner the bigoudi should be, to obtain a tighter roll under.

Be certain that the hair is thoroughly dry before removing the hair pins.

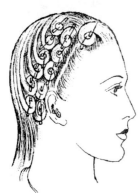

Fig. 123.

Place half wave in first Basic No. 8, commence curling from the top.

The Dressing Out

As in most dressings, back-combing is essential to create fullness and height. Comb the front curls through, back-comb underneath, smooth the top and place in position with the curl on the hair line as shown in finished picture, Fig. 127. Comb all the hair through at back and sides. Should a fuller effect be required, then back-comb the underneath part. A smoother effect can be obtained by dividing a portion of the top hair, and, after the underneath hair has been back-combed, combing all the hair down; this method will give you a smoother finish. The sides, being a half-wave movement, should be combed up high. The completed dressing as illustrated portrays an elegant movement, shows the natural shape of the head and gives an elongated effect. The C curl on the small side is dressed-out separately, back-combed to make it fuller and allowing the curl also to fall on the hair line giving the completed dressing a perfect line of symmetry.

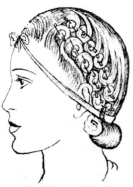

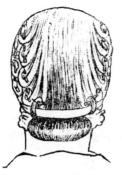

Fig. 124. Ribbon is placed securely at the nape, over the ears and tied in the front. A large curl on each side is pinned over the tape.

Fig. 125. Hair is rolled under over a crepe bigoudi and pinned securely.

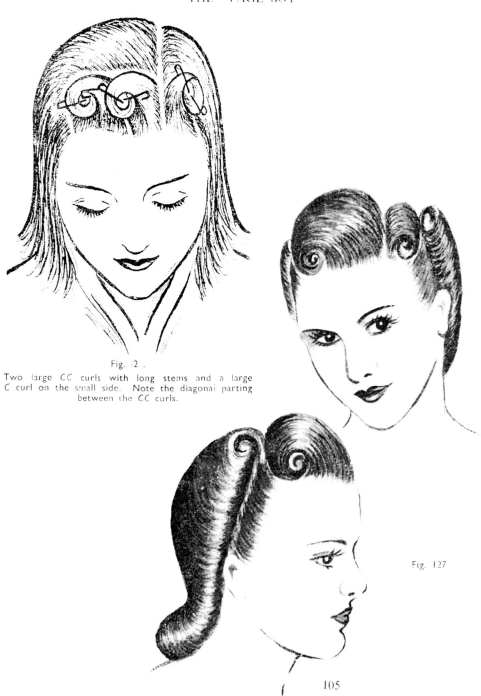

Fig. 12.
Two large CC curls with long stems and a large
C curl on the small side. Note the diagonal parting
between the CC curls.

Fig. 127

105

"Page Boy" Variations

LIKE most designs, varying the pli in the "Page Boy" will present a different movement for the completed dressing. You should have in mind before starting the correct design—for example, length, width, towards the face, off the face, the movement for the sides, swirls, waves, curls or a half-wave. All these movements carefully thought out before beginning the pli play an important part, and your dressing out problems will be comparatively easier.

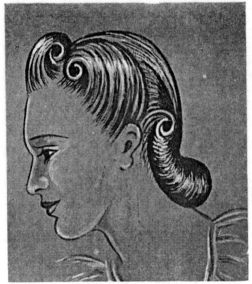

Fig. 128.

Fig. 128 presents a variation of the "Page Boy." The sides have a swirled movement; the "Page Boy" is combed towards the centre. In Figs. 123 and 124 the back hair is combed towards the face, but the pli of Fig. 129 clearly shows the back hair combed in a circular movement towards the centre of the back, and when this pli is dressed-out the back appears narrower than if the hair was combed towards the face.

Another design could be made from this dressing by joining together with a slide the curls on each side, or by placing a ribbon under the "Page Boy," joining the ends together and making a bow. The effect at the back would be that of a "Page Boy" bun.

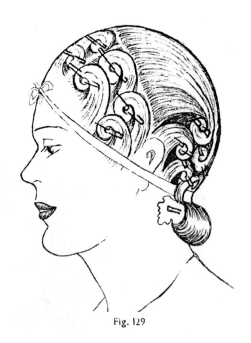

Fig. 129. The back hair is well shaped from the sides towards the centre.

Fig. 129

106

Fig. 130 is another variation. The hair is placed in pli well forward, and when dressed-out will cover the ear. The roll-under will be well to the face. The side sweep must be dressed-out first so that the "Page Boy" sides can be pinned over it.

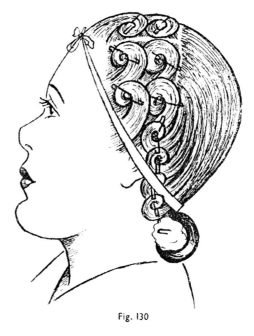

Fig. 130

Fig. 130. The sides are brought well forward. The side swirls are Basic No. 10.

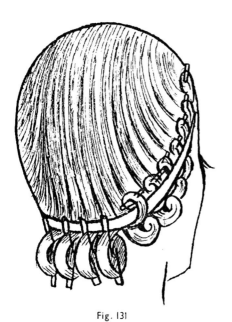

Fig. 131

Fig. 131. A large curl is pinned over the tape on each side. The rolled under curls are held securely by inserting a pin upward and another downward.

Fig. 131 shows a pli variation; instead of a crepe bigoudi being used, the curls are rolled under. I find this method useful when the hair is thick and curly; furthermore, the hair does not take so long to dry. Care must be taken when placing the net over, to avoid flattening the curls.

Fig. 132 is another example of a "Page Boy" dressing: instead of a roll-under movement, it has a wave across. This wave is obtained by curling the ends on a bigoudi as shown in Fig. 133. Should the hair be very thick, then two layers of curls can be made on the reverse curl method. This would also make a more definite wave. Pinning the curls on the crepe roll will ensure that the dressing will stand away from the groove made by the tape. My adaption of the "Page Boy" dressing will, with practice, give you infinite scope to vary and modify your own creations to suit the individual.

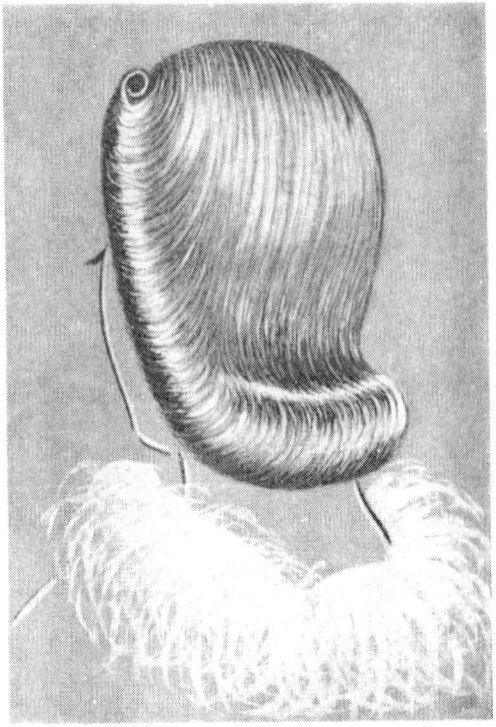

Fig. 132.

'Page Boy" design showing wave under roll.

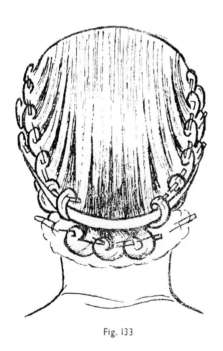

Fig. 133

Fig. 133. By pinning the curls close to the tape the crest of the wave will be accentuated.

CHAPTER TWENTY-ONE

Hair Style Designs "Très Chic." (Fig. 134)

THE creation of a style must be based on a set plan, basically prepared and scientifically produced. Once you have decided on the lay-out of a suggested style you have in mind, then the basic principles lay the foundation. First, observe the complete dressing. Here you will notice the side front movement. You will recognise it as Basic No. 6. The ability to visualise artistically the proper lay-out of the style stimulates the imagination. Although this dressing may seem to be rather complicated, it can be carried out even by the student.

Setting Instructions

The movement combed well up off the hair line and forming the basic principle No. 6 is the predominating feature of the "Très Chic" design. Place the curls as shown in the sketch, Fig. 135. Six C curls over the first complete wave. The right side has a small movement as the lower position of basic No. 7, the curls finishing in CC direction. The rest of the hair on top is also curled in the same CC direction, well forward to the front.

Although the back may seem complicated to a student, it is in fact a simple pattern. As quite a lot of hair has been taken up from the back for the side movement, there remains little hair for the back. Make a diagonal parting from the left side, about two inches from the hair line, extended to the nape.

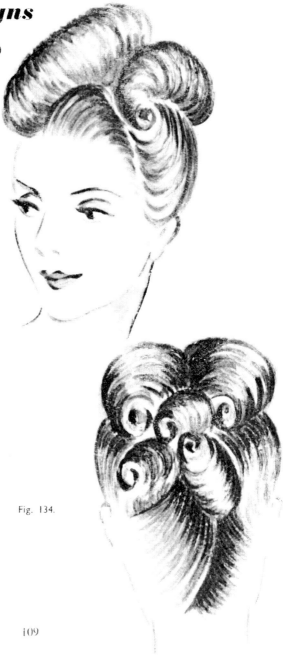

Fig. 134.

109

Comb the hair from the right side towards the extreme left, placing the ends in *CC* curls. Cross the hair from the left side, overlapping as shown in sketch, and finishing in *C* curls.

The Dressing Out

The art of combing to achieve a desired effect cannot be learned in a few lessons. Constant practice will, however, inspire confidence in students and make them creative stylists.

You must have a mental picture of the general *ensemble* you wish to achieve. Should the shape not be to your artistic liking, then re-comb until you are satisfied.

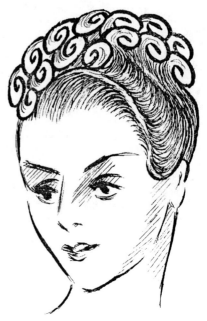

Fig. 135. Front wave basic No. 6 with 6 large C curls over crest. Right side similar positions but smaller and set in CC curls

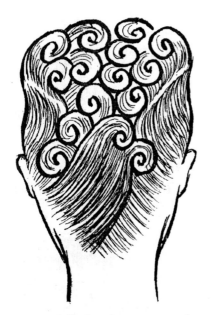

Fig. 136. Comb back into position right side just after making a diagonal parting

"Très-Chic" dressing should not present much difficulty if the pli is correctly placed. The left side should be the first movement to be combed out. Comb well through, lift the hair well up and back-comb on the inside; smooth the top hair and place a side comb above the wave, allowing the top hair to roll forward. The same procedure for the right side, but with extra back-combing to create a larger movement coming forward with a side comb inserted fairly high to produce a higher effect. The back design is dressed out in the same manner as the pli. The hair that is combed over from the left side must be smooth; insert a comb, pushing up slightly to form a slight wave movement.

"Soignée" Fig. 137

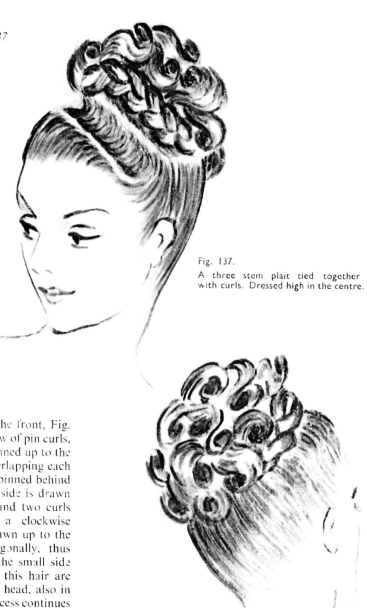

THIS dressing is simple, easy to accomplish, graceful and becoming. There is an increasing demand for the upward trend of hair styling, arranged and dressed off the face. This style is suitable for the person who is tall and striking, and whose face is oblong or oval.

Grecian sculpture is a classic example of this style. To model our hairdressing on the designs of immortal paintings and sculpture gives us endless opportunities to renew the artistic interpretations of those masters. I have called this style "Soignée" because I think it embodies the artistic conceptions of the masters.

Fig. 137.
A three stem plait tied together with curls. Dressed high in the centre.

Setting Instructions

A full wave is formed in the front, Fig. 138, slightly on a slant, and a row of pin curls, comprising three in a row, is pinned up to the last ridge, each curl slightly overlapping each other. Another row of curls is pinned behind this one. The hair on the left side is drawn up, and away from the face, and two curls are pinned horizontally, in a clockwise direction. The back hair is drawn up to the crown, Fig. 139, slightly diagonally, thus ensuring the hair going from the small side into the big side; the ends of this hair are pin-curled on to the top of the head, also in a clockwise direction. This process continues

111

HAIR STYLE DESIGNS

"Soignée"

right round to the right hand side of the head. There is no main parting in this dressing.

Dressing Out

A three stem plait is made from a switch, the ends of which are tied together, thereby forming a plaited loop of the required size, to sit on the crown of the head. The hair is all combed upwards, the curls combed through together, and the wave smoothed into position. The plaited loop is placed over the hair and pinned securely to the head, and the hair drawn through it. The ends are now combed out, back-combed, smoothed and dressed by the reverse curl method into flat waved curls, arranged in the centre of the plait.

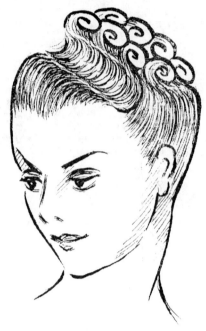

Fig. 138. A complete slanting wave, with two rows of C curls.

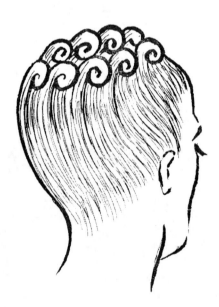

Fig. 139. Hair combed diagonally with C curls on crown.

112

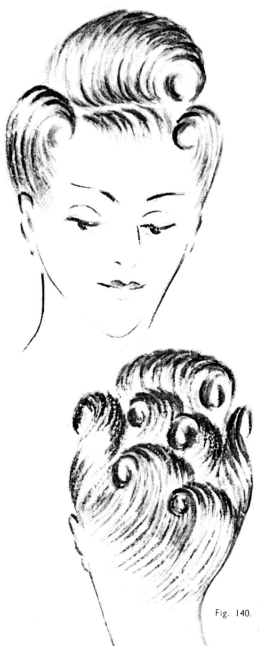

"Prestige" *Fig. 140.*

ITS versatility makes short hair a favour-ite fashion. The accomplishment of skilful work depends on the accuracy of hair preparation in the important *foundation of tapering.* All the explanation of practical and elaborate styles is futile unless the hair is prepared accordingly. Enormous possibilities are at your disposal. And to satisfy the demands of your clients for exclusive coiffures, you must realise that pliability of tapered hair is the secret of success. To achieve the best results with the style which I have called "Prestige," you must pay the same careful attention to preparation.

Setting Instructions

The hair is parted on the left side, Fig. 141, and a half-wave set into position, Basic No. 1. Three curls are pinned up to this ridge, overlapping each other slightly, with the curl farthest from the parting having the longest stem, to ensure a good shape to the swirl. Another similar row of curls is set behind this row. A slightly slanted parting is taken, each side, to just behind each ear, and these front pieces are left to be set up last of all. Beginning on the right side of the back, Fig. 142, the hair is pinned into swirl curls, which have slanting partings for their bases, the stems being taken from left to right, and the curls going upwards towards the crown of the head, so that the whole formation of the back is slanting slightly from the small side into the big side and all the swirl curls overlap each other's stems. The sides are now pinned into four swirl curls each, the first row covering the partings. Basic No. 10.

Fig. 140.

"Prestige"

Dressing Out

Front. The back three curls of the front are combed right out, and held taut with the left hand. The strand is back-combed extensively at the roots, and lightly to the ends, on the top surface, while simultaneously the left hand moves the strand backwards. The half-wave and remaining three curls are back-combed similarly, except that this time the back-combing is done on the under surface of the strand. The operator now stands behind the head, smooths both strands together and backwards, with a postiche brush or comb, and then, starting at the ends, rolls the hair under. The half-wave is gently replaced, and

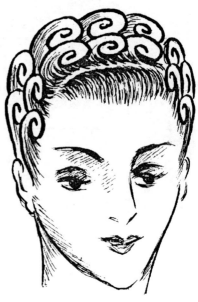

Fig. 141. A half wave as in Basic No. 1, with two rows of C curls. Sides as in Basic No. 10.

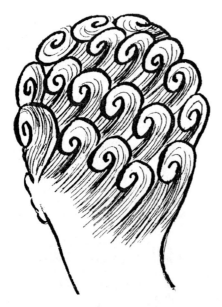

Fig. 142. Make two partings diagonally from the right side extending to the crown. Long stem CC swirled curls made in formation.

the swirl held flat between the palms of the hands, and pressed to make the wave fall in deeply. This top half-waved swirl is now pinned into position. The back is separated into four larger portions, each portion having a slanting parting at its base, and incorporating several curls. The top swirled curl is the first to do. It is back-combed at the roots and lightly to the ends, on the under surface, smoothed, and formed into a large swirl going towards the crown. The remaining three portions are arranged similarly, each one covering the preceding partings. A little lacquer sprayed on the back curls would keep them in position more securely. The four curls at the sides are now dressed also into swirls, in the same way, and cover the side partings. A comb may be used for the back if necessary. It forms a decoration and assists in keeping the hair in position.

114

"*Magnifique*" Fig. 143.

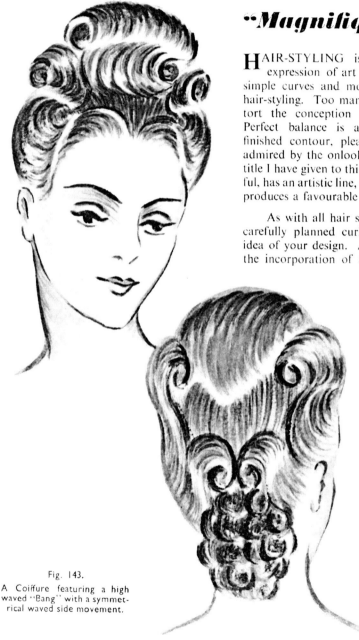

HAIR-STYLING is principally a graceful expression of art and rhythm. Sometimes simple curves and movements predominate in hair-styling. Too many ideas on one head distort the conception and create disharmony. Perfect balance is always expressed in the finished contour, pleasing to the wearer and admired by the onlooker. "Magnifique" is the title I have given to this style, because it is graceful, has an artistic line, creates height, and always produces a favourable reaction.

As with all hair styles, the arrangement of carefully planned curls will produce the final idea of your design. As previously mentioned, the incorporation of a number of movements placed together will evolve a nice conception. This dressing is composed of a number of movements collected from different designs. The back design was demonstrated by me in Denmark on one of my coiffures. The front movement is a predominating fashion on the Continent. Much of the success of a hairdress depends on how the style reacts in shape on the individual.

Setting Instructions

Study the pli formation on the accompanying sketch. Comb the hair straight back from the forehead. Make a V parting from the centre of the front. Allow the side

Fig. 143.
A Coiffure featuring a high waved "Bang" with a symmetrical waved side movement.

115

hair to hang away from the partings, while the hair within the V shape is placed in *C* curls as in Fig. 144. Make another V parting at the back as in Fig. 145 and place into *C* curls as shown. The back hair is combed down and a portion is taken off at each side. These are done after the hair at the nape is curled. This curling is done by dividing the hair in the centre, *C* curls on the left side, and *CC* curls on the right side.

The hair at the sides of the neck has a long stem formed into curls pushed up slightly into a half-waved movement which will fall towards the centre. From the centre of the front, form an upward movement and place a front crest as in Basic No. 11. After this crest, drag the hair well up to form a large waved movement, as shown, with curls close up to the ridge.

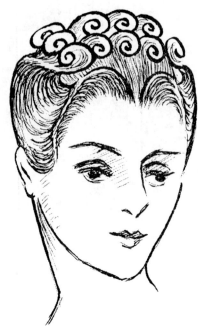

Fig. 144. Complete centre *C* curls in V parting, with side movement overlapping.

The Dressing Out

As "Magnifique" is a high dressing, it is essential that the back-combing is done close to the scalp, not near the front, as this part is kept straight. Comb all the top curls together, make a parting across the top near to the V shape at the back, back-comb the roots, make another parting, and repeat the back-combing. Then hold all the top hair together, back-comb the roots about half-way across the head, brush the hair smoothly over the palm of the hand, and, with the comb, shape a wave, gently removing the left hand. Pin the waves temporarily until the dressing is completed. Next, complete the back, dressing the curls at the nape first, then back-comb the upward curls and pin securely. The sides must be well combed out. Place a side comb above the crest or securely fasten with grips. Spray a little lacquer over the completed dressing.

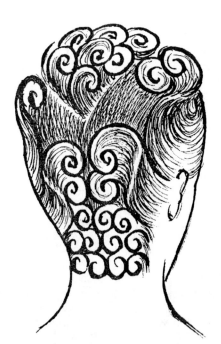

Fig. 145. V parting curls extended to crown. Hair smoothed down with overlapping movement at sides.

116

"Aspiration"

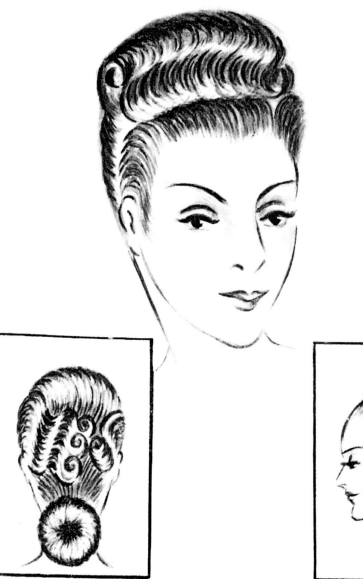

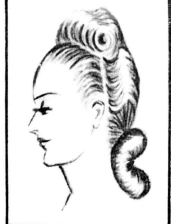

Fig. 146.

HAIR STYLE DESIGNS

"Aspiration"   Fig. 146.

THIS coiffure, originally created for formal occasions, can easily be arranged in a more simple pattern. This style is therefore practical and flattering, and provides an important opportunity for the student to practise the technicalities already explained. Thus the possibility of variation is limitless.

This design shows two methods of curling, the stand-up curls for the front, and the bigoudi curls for the back. The frontal technique can be varied for a waved bang, rolled bang, forward roll, fluffy curled front, and many other designs. The bigoudi curls can be dressed out with loose curls, large puff curls, a doughnut design, ringlets and numerous others.

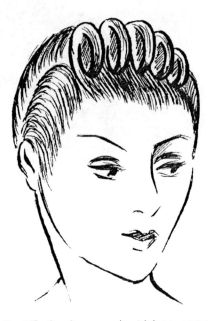

Setting Instructions

Part off the amount of hair required for the front curls, Fig. 147. Place as many standing up curls as necessary for the amount of wave required Larger curls will produce larger waves; tighter curls will make deeper waves with curled ends. For this design, being a flat front wave, large

Fig. 147. Standing up curls with large centres forming top movement.

curls are made. The side movement is taken into an upward wave, Fig. 148, the crest falling behind the ear. The large side is extended into waves across the back, Fig. 149, finishing off with large flat curls. The small side has one crest behind the ear, finishing off with a large flat curl. Should the hair be thick, then more curls can be made.

So that the hair on the crown does not show too flat, large curls are placed which can be dressed out separately, or combed with the front curls, as shown in the completed picture. The rest of the hair is combed to the centre of the nape and rolled on paper or crepe bigoudis. Do not have the hair too wet when curling; so long as there is a little dampness the hair will curl quite tightly.

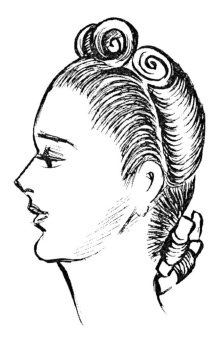

Fig. 148. An upward wave is made with the crest falling behind the ear.

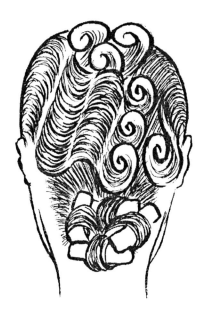

Fig. 149. Hair at nape drawn towards centre placed into elastic band, curls rolled on bigoudis.

The Dressing Out

Comb through the front curls, part off in divisions, and well back-comb at the roots, keeping the hair back. Brush over the palm of the hand to ensure smoothness, and gently push into waves. Place hairpins in the centre of the waves, and do not remove until the entire dressing is completed. Separate the side movements, and comb the rest of the hair down to the centre of the nape. Place all the hair in a small elastic band. Comb the hair into position from the centre, back-comb in sections and roll over. It is advisable to place an invisible net over the doughnut dressing. To create a fullness on the side movement, back-comb underneath and spread out if required. A larger "doughnut" can be made by combing the hair over a crepe pad.

119

"*Harmony*" Fig. 150

THIS simple and practical design, which should prove very useful in general saloon use, is built on a perfect symmetry. The length of hair for the front should be 8 to 10 inches long. The balance of this hairdressing is an important feature. The waves must be in the correct angle, off the face, exposing the hair line, with the exception of the slight dip in front. The back favours an Edwardian movement, quite simple to carry out.

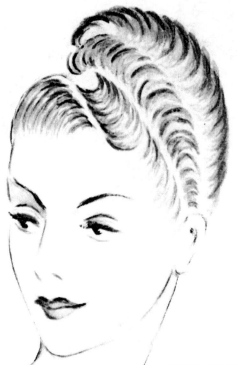

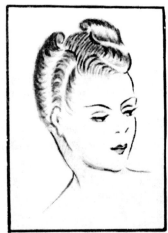

Fig. 150.

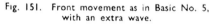

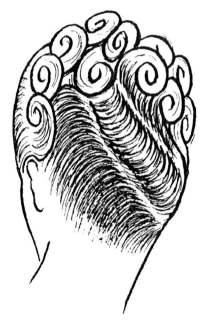

Fig. 151. Front movement as in Basic No. 5, with an extra wave.

Fig. 152. Two large swirled CC curls with upward and downward stem.

Setting Instructions

This dressing, Fig. 151, is on the principle of Basic No. 5, with an extra wave. The importance of combing the hair towards the parting cannot be over-emphasised, as this movement tends to lift the dressing to its desired shape. By studying the accompanying sketch, Fig. 151, you will notice that the hair is well off the face in front of the ear, so that a downward wave is the first movement on the hair line. Keep the elbow well up when doing the right side and the elbow well down when setting the left side (this does not apply to left handed setters). Follow carefully the position of the placing of the curls. Two large *CC* curls are placed in position on the back of the crown, the upper one with the stem going upwards and the lower with stem combed downwards, as in Fig. 152. These curls are dressed out separately as shown in the miniature completed dressing. The back is swathed upwards, waved on a slant, finishing with large curls which can be dressed out separately or combed into large movements.

The Dressing Out

This dressing, being practical, will lend itself to plenty of combing. Begin on the large side of the front, comb well through, divide in sections, and back-comb at the roots, as this dressing should be high. No back-combing will keep the hair flat and mar the shape. Back-comb to the ends and brush over carefully. The order of the combing of each individual portion of hair is identical to that of its formation, the large side first, the small side, and then the back. The completed drawing shows the side movements dressed high, sleek top from the parting and the back dressed out into large curls.

121

Hair Styles For All

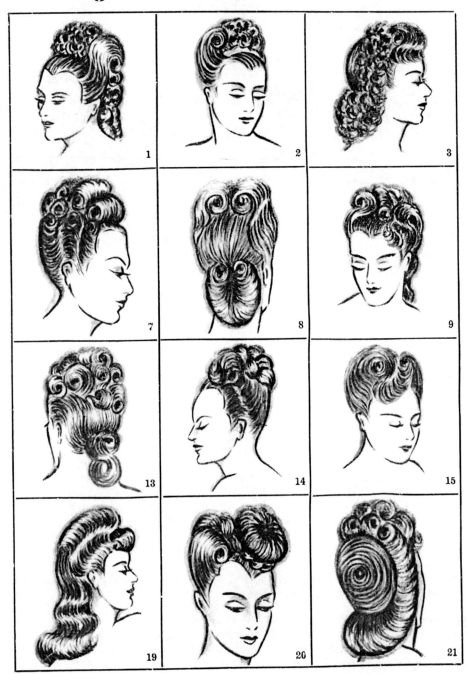

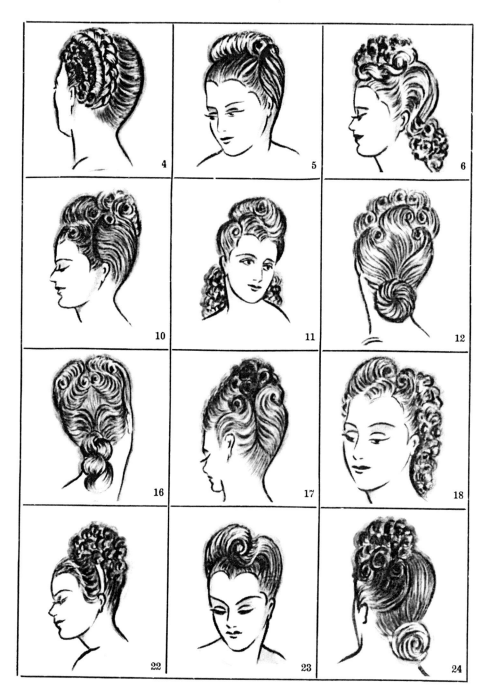

4

5

6

10

11

12

16

17

18

22

23

24

123

"Olympia" *Fig. 153*

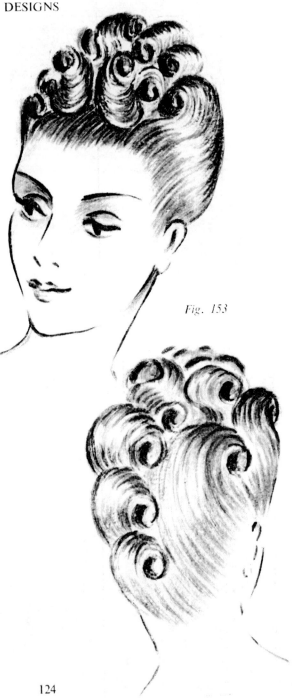

Fig. 153

*C*REATIVE *Hair Styling* is your professional guide. It is designed to keep you *au fait* with improvements in service techniques, and to introduce to you a simple narration of technical knowledge which will contribute to your success and develop your professional prestige.

Although the "Olympia" style may seem at first to be beyond your skill, you will find that it is more simple than it looks. Always take advantage of an opportunity to carry out a different design and be prepared to undertake skilfully any style that appeals to your clients.

I have called this design "Olympia" because it was acclaimed to be more outstanding than all the dressings I exhibited at the *Daily Mail* Ideal Home Exhibition, Olympia, in 1947. This design offers unlimited possibilities and a new trend in simplicity. The hair is brushed clear from the forehead and the sleek upswept lines produce an effect of classic charm.

Setting Instructions

The top hair should not be longer than four to six inches. Beginning at the front, Fig. 154, make long *C* curls on the right side and long *CC* curls on the left side. Make a second row, also placed in the same direction, and close to the first curls. Divide the hair on each side from the top curls to the back of the ear, leave the pli of the sides till last. The back hair is curled in long stems towards

124

one side, Fig. 155. Make the partings for these curls in a diagonal movement. So that the curls do not fall down, place a hair pin from the top of the curl downwards. Now comb the sides into position, making an upward movement, only one crest, and the ends curled immediately behind.

The Dressing Out

Although the design in the pli formation sketch shows a centre parting, and the sketch for the completed dressing shows no parting, this is optional. There is a tendency for the parting to show because the curls are placed in opposite directions. To avoid this, if the parting is not required, place a small slide or comb in the centre, which becomes covered by the top hair. The curls on top are combed out loose. The ends are formed

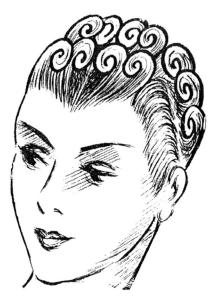

Fig. 154. Centre parting
with long stem curls.

into a wave on each side towards the centre, loose curls are immediately behind, and large puff curls placed on the crown. These puff curls come from the back curls near the crown. Complete the back before the sides. Make a long diagonal parting at the back which would take up about four large curls on the right side, comb the curls together, and make a large swirled movement. With the remaining hair on the left side, make two diagonal partings, back-comb each section, and dress into flat swirled puff curls. Now complete the side movements. Comb well through, make diagonal partings, well back-comb the roots and the whole of the hair, then hold the whole of the side together, back-comb again, brush smoothly tucking the ends well under. The effect is a long waved sweep. If well done, this dressing will reflect credit on you. Constant practice with this style, to overcome any difficulties, will subsequently repay you for the time spent.

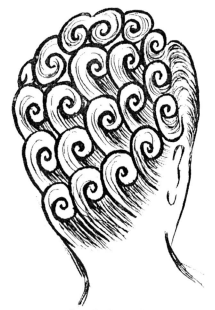

Fig. 155. Diagonal.
Based swirled curls.

The "Bolster Roll" Fig. 156

THIS coiffure is similar to the "Aspiration" design, and the front movement is based on the same line. I have designed this dressing for practical purposes, and it is one which can be carried out even by the novice. The practice of this dressing will help considerably to vary delightful adaptations for day and evening wear.

Here is a perfect example of the basic principles. The front movement is Basic No. 1, the sides Basic No. 9, incorporating a swathed Edwardian for the back dressing. It is reasonably easy to keep in position, is essentially an up-to-date style, and as a saloon dressing it would be hard to surpass.

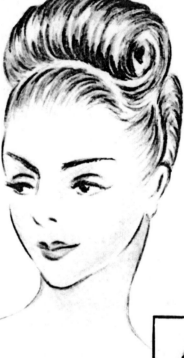

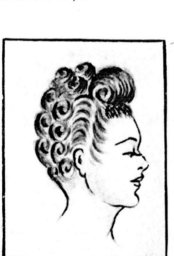

Fig. 156

HAIR STYLE DESIGNS

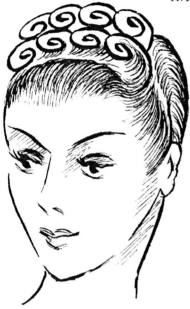

Fig. 157. Front as Basic No. 1.

Setting Instructions

Every dressing should be carried out with scrupulous care. By observing Fig. 157 carefully, you will notice that, as in Basic No. 1, the hair is well shaped on the hair line, and two rows of curls are immediately behind the sharp crest. The side movement, Fig. 158, should be done next, which is Basic No. 9. Copy the wave and curls as shown for the back, Fig. 159.

The Dressing Out

The order of combing is similar to that of the pli. Comb out the two rows of curls of the front and well back-comb on the top of the hair to produce a large puff roll. The sides also must be well combed out, separating the curls or making a large movement, but these should be done after the back has been dressed out. The back dressing, which is an Edwardian, must be kept up by using combs or grips. All short hairs which may have a tendency to separate must be brushed smoothly. A little lacquer or pomade, well-brushed, will keep up the ends.

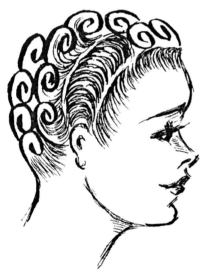

Fig. 158. Sides as in Basic No. 9.

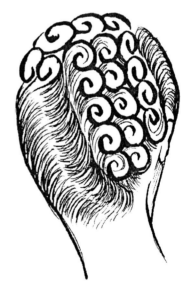

Fig. 159 A slightly off-vertical wave with two rows of C curls.

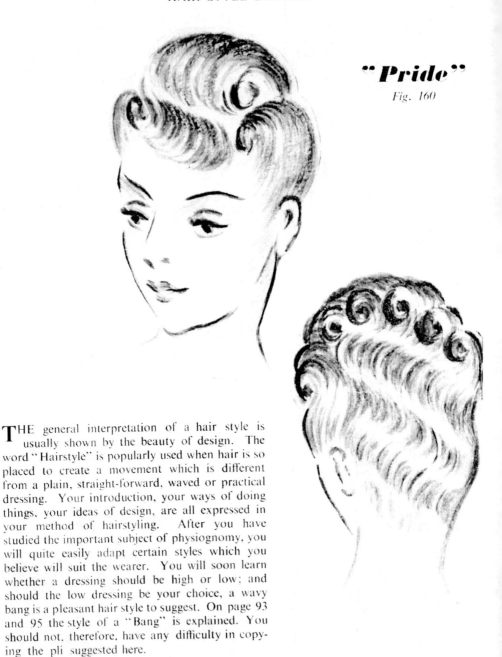

"Pride"

Fig. 160

THE general interpretation of a hair style is usually shown by the beauty of design. The word "Hairstyle" is popularly used when hair is so placed to create a movement which is different from a plain, straight-forward, waved or practical dressing. Your introduction, your ways of doing things, your ideas of design, are all expressed in your method of hairstyling. After you have studied the important subject of physiognomy, you will quite easily adapt certain styles which you believe will suit the wearer. You will soon learn whether a dressing should be high or low; and should the low dressing be your choice, a wavy bang is a pleasant hair style to suggest. On page 93 and 95 the style of a "Bang" is explained. You should not, therefore, have any difficulty in copying the pli suggested here.

128

HAIR STYLE DESIGNS

Setting Instructions

Divide the hair near the crown and make an even side parting, Fig. 161. Two rows of curls extended backward off the hair line. Make a division from the side parting to the back of the ear. Leave the side curls until you have completed the back effect, which is an Edwardian dressing with diagonal waves, Fig. 162. The ends are finished off with curls. The side movement placed in swirl curls is Basic No. 10.

The Dressing Out

The top curls are combed well out. Begin with a parting across the hair line,

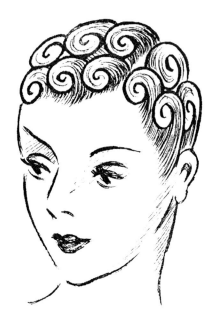

Fig. 161. Make a parting on each side. Top curls are all CC . Sides Basic No. 10.

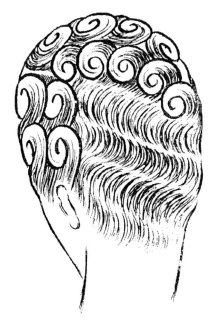

Fig. 162. Complete the back pli before the side swirls.

back-comb down to the scalp to create a little height, repeat the divisions and back-comb. Stand in the front of your client, brush smoothly over your left hand, and form a wave with the comb. Pins will keep the waves in position until the dressing is completed. The back movement should be combed out next, as the side swirls should overlap the parting. The curls at the back can be dressed either in separate curls or a large movement combed all in one. Should the side swirls be desired dressed high, then more back-combing well down at the roots must be made.

129

"Soir de Bal" *Fig. 163*

THE title of this dressing suggests that it is intended for a big occasion. The design will appeal to your client who wants something which is outstanding but simple to carry out. The predominating feature of the ensemble is that the hairdresser can modify the design or vary the shape; it provides many opportunities for artistic expression.

Setting Instructions

Front. Fig. 164. A side parting is made on the right side. The hair is then combed back and across the front of the head, away from the parting, formed into a crest, based on the position of the first wave in a two-wave set off the face. Three large *CC* curls are pinned into position into this crest, beginning with the back curl so that the consecutive curls can overlap each other slightly. Another row, comprising two *C* pin-curls, is made behind the first row.

Partings from the side swirls are now made from the crown to just behind the ear, and these sections of hair left to be pinned after the back hair has been placed en pli.

Back. Fig. 165. A curved parting is made, beginning at the top of the ear on the right side, and extending upwards to the centre of the crown; the hair above this parting is placed out of the way, to be set later on. This portion must be cut shorter than the underneath

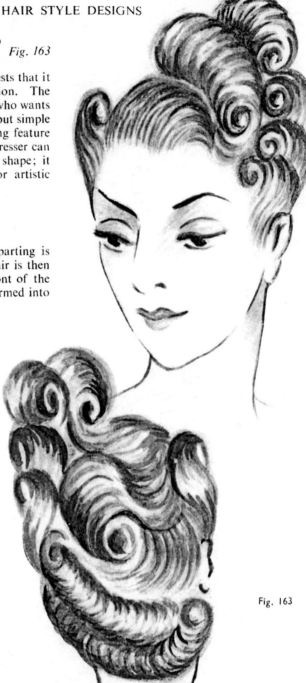

Fig. 163

130

hair. The remaining hair at the back is swept downwards and across to the left side, and formed into a circular crest. A row of *CC* curls is pinned up to this crest, with a similar row underneath.

Now the loose hair on the top is combed downwards and across, and formed into a smaller crest, which follows the lower one in all particulars, and is exactly parallel to it. The curls are similar, but are pinned over the flat part of the lower hair, so that the top curls overlap the lower movement.

The back now being completed, the side pieces are placed en pli. The left side is divided into three large swirl curls, one behind the other, the one nearest the face having a lightly waved movement in it. The right side is set into two similar swirl curls.

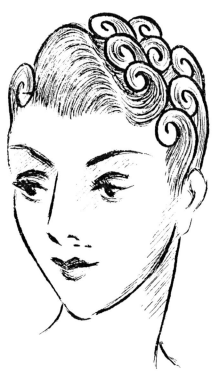

Fig. 164. Hair must be taken well off the front. A diagonal wave and a larger stretched front curl.

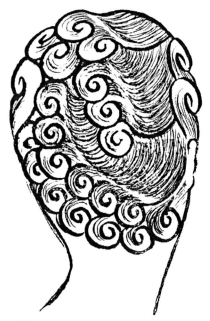

Fig. 165. The front side curls are completed after the back pli. A curved parting is made from the right ear extending upwards to the centre of the crown.

The Dressing Out

The front three curls are combed through together. The operator stands at the left side of the client and holds this strand taut with the left hand, while back-combing it with the right hand, on the top surface.

The strand is then rolled forward so that the back-combing is inside, and the top hair is smoothed and formed into a large rolled cockscomb across the top of the head. The two *CC* curls are back-combed underneath, and another roll, which will fall in the opposite direction to the previous one, is formed in the same way.

131

HAIR STYLE DESIGNS

The lower section at the back is now dressed as it was put en pli, the first row of curls back-combed on the top surface, and placed into a large roll sitting under the crest. The second row of curls will form another similar roll underneath this one.

The top section at the back is back-combed underneath and smoothed on the top. The ends are rolled under to form a large waved swirl, finishing with a curl fitting into the curve of the lower hair.

The left side is combed into three separate swirls, each one being back-combed on the under surface, and smoothed upwards and placed into position. The two curls on the right side are either combed together into one large swirl movement, or can be divided and dressed into two swirl curls corresponding with the two lower curls on the left side. A little lacquer sprayed on the hair will help to keep the dressing in position. Comb or flower ornaments added to this dressing will create a graceful interpretation of hair artistry.

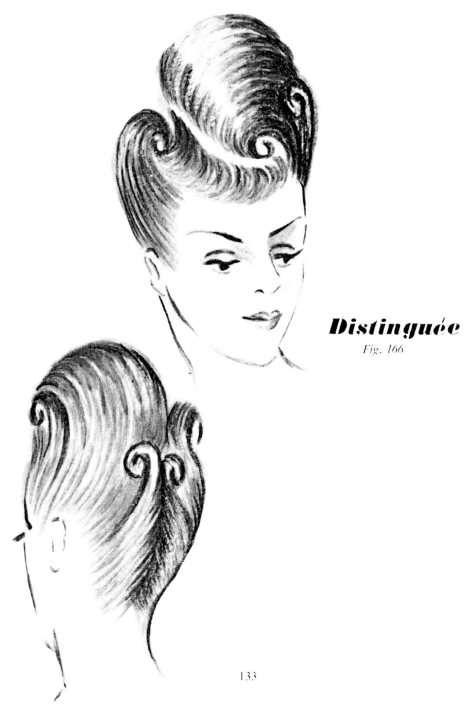

Distinguée

Fig. 166

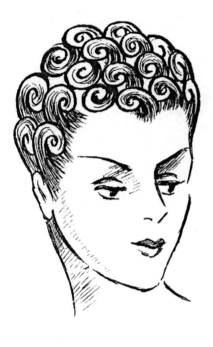

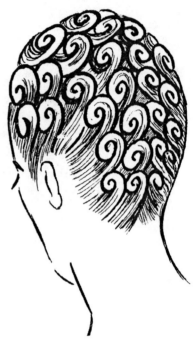

Fig. 167. The three C curls reversed to the top curls will make a deeper front wave.

Fig. 168. A centre parting at back with curls placed in pli towards the parting with long stems.

Distinguée *Fig. 166*

MANY hairdressers believe that intricate hair arrangements can be achieved only by specialist stylists; on the contrary, every hairdresser can carry out a dressing if certain fundamentals are adopted, and certain rules respected: Study proportion, create harmonious line, follow the pendulum of fashion. The use of the correct technique creates confidence in every student or experienced hairdresser, gives personal pleasure and satisfaction, for our craft cannot be pursued unless it is inspired by genuine interest. The designs in this book are thoroughly practical, can be created and copied in the saloon, modified or adapted to any design that may suit your client's features, so that the entire ensemble expresses gracefulness.

This particular coiffure has a pronounced distinguished appearance. The introduction of a new or distinctive style always increases your prestige as a hair stylist. The woman who wears her hair in this "Distinguée" design, does so with a sense of drama and imagination. Providing the features and "Distinguée" harmonise, there will be an atmosphere of elegance and dramatic glamour. Before the pli is begun, the hair for the bang movement *must* be tapered to the correct length.

134

HAIR STYLE DESIGNS

Setting Instructions. Fig. 167

The high upswept movement is on the left side. Separate the right side where the four large swirled curls are shown, make a parting from the front to the crown and place three large *C* curls each in its own base without a stem. The remaining hair is all placed in *CC* swirled curls with a stem. The hair on the right side is an arrangement of *C* curls with a long stem. Make a centre parting at the back, Fig. 168. Divide each side again, beginning near the centre parting, *CC* curls on the left side and *C* curls on the right, all having long stems. Place a hairpin on the top of the curl going downwards, so that the curls are kept up securely.

The Dressing Out

This coiffure is a remarkable example of dressing-out technique for it involves great skill in execution. Remove the hair on the right side, also a small portion for a large swirl for the left side. Comb the rest of the hair on top together. Make a diagonal parting from left to right near the hair line. Lift up and back-comb at the roots, continue making diagonal partings until all the hair is back-combed. As this is a high dressing, it is essential that the back-combing is done right down to the roots, to make the rest of the hair stand upright. Take all the hair together in the left hand on a slant, brush the hair smoothly; you will then find that the wave can easily be placed into the desired position as shown. Place pins in the crest to keep the wave in position. Continue with the large side swirl. The large swirl on the right side interlocks the curls from the end of the waved bang movement. Many variations can be made from the pli of "Distinguée," and can be ornamented to give distinguished and artistic expressions of Hair Beauty.

135

Variation of Hair Styles created
Daily Mail Ideal Home

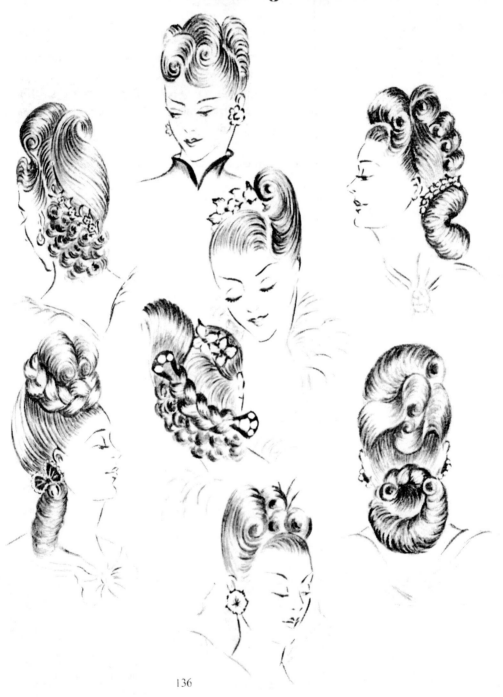

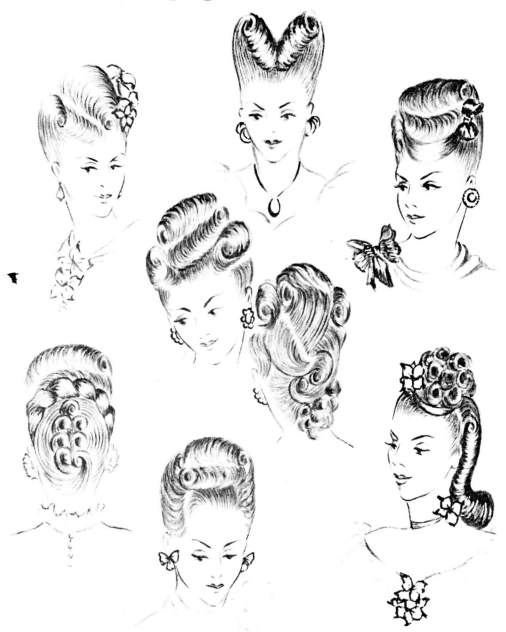

CHAPTER TWENTY-TWO

Modern Hair Fashions Influenced By Historical Hairdressing

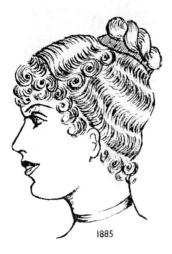

1885

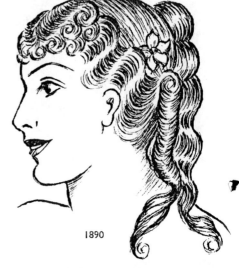

1890

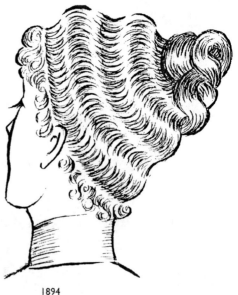

1894

WOMEN have always been hair-conscious. As I have said in a previous chapter, most of our inspirations for modern hair dressing are based on ideas passed down through the ages. Beautifying the hair was as important to our ancestors as it is to us. A luxuriant and historic coiffure portrays an example of real hair artistry, and to-day our designers have taken a movement from one historical dressing, combined it with a movement from another, and thus created a modern style. The accompanying illustrations will show you how ancient hair styling has been brought up-to-date.

Let us trace the origin of some of our modern styles and ways of hairdressing.

In the time of the Pharaohs, the ancient Egyptians used the same hennas to tint the

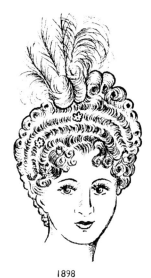

1898

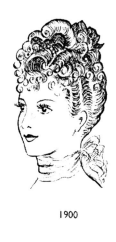

1900

hair as we do to-day. They also devised a method of permanent waving by winding meshes of hair, dipped in solution, on crude sticks, allowing these to dry in the sun and eventually achieving a crimpiness in the hair, which was the prevailing fashion. Egyptian women of high rank took infinite pains with their hair, and the fashion was to wear the hair in a fringe across the forehead, either in the form of flat curls, or in a heavy fall of "crimped" hair on the brow, presumably their nearest approach to obtaining the wavy hair which women have desired from time immemorial!

Thus the fringes and "bangs" of to-day are not original, although by interpreting them in different ways we obtain some very attractive modern versions of them.

Hairdressing, like all other great Arts, is international, and we find a little of all nations in our present hair styling. The plaits we include now must surely have emanated from the Chinese, to whom the "pigtail" worn by the men was a form of religion, and who considered its removal to bring the greatest ignominy.

A London fashion of 1921-1922 was that of having the hair coiled over the ears to form "ear-phones." This was rather a striking adaptation of the Geisha girls' coiffure of Japan, though, fortunately, it did not necessitate the use of special neck supports at night to keep it in position, as was customary in that country.

Spain has also contributed to the art of hair-styling. The dark luxuriant heads of the Senoritas with their beautiful coils and chignons were indeed an inspiration to other countries. Now that glossy coils are again fashionable, many modern hair stylists would be grateful to know the secret of the old Spanish art of making glossy coils.

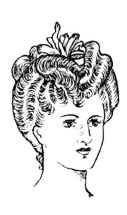

1903

It is strange to find that to-day we still have traces of the Medieval. One of the most popular modern styles has been the "Page Boy," which again can only be classed as a modern adaptation of the haircut given to small boys attending the medieval knights of old at Court.

One of the most sophisticated styles of to-day is that of the "doughnut" perched on the crown of the head with the

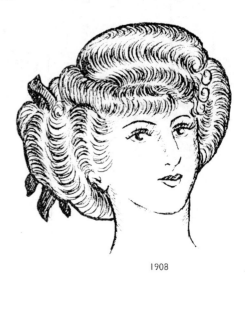

1908

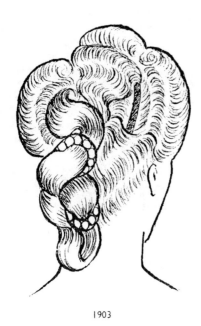

1903

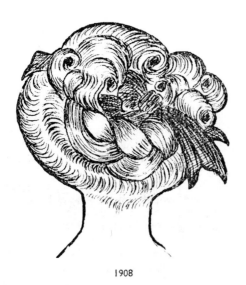

1908

rest of the hair being drawn up to it. A "Soignée" coiffure, it is very similar to that worn by the ladies of Siam.

The oldest hair style in the world— and yet the youngest—is the short "bubble" cut, so recently popular. Babies with their curly hair beginning to grow all over their heads, must surely have inspired this modern form of coiffure.

Even the substances we use to-day to enhance the hair are only improvements on earlier methods. Oils, pomades, creams and perfumes were all used by the Egyptians, Chinese, Romans, and so on. We keep a coiffure neatly in place by spraying lacquer over it, while the most primitive ancient and modern African tribes mix clay in their hair when dressing it to keep it in position.

Ancient Greece has, I consider, con-tributed most to the art of hairdressing. The Greeks had a fetish for purity of line,

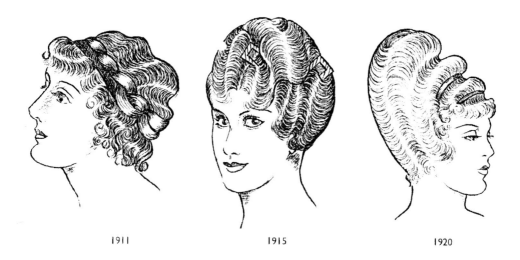

1911   1915   1920

harmony and balance in all their works of art, and they incorporated all these in their hair styling. They did not aim to create elaborate coiffures, but those which suited the shape of the head, the features of the face, the line of the neck and shoulders, and the physique of the body—in fact the *tout ensemble*.

Their study of physiognomy is an example to any hairdresser of to-day. We may create the most becoming and original hair style, but it can never be perfect if we have not the skill to make it to suit the features and form of the person for whom it is created.

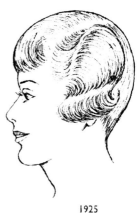

1925

141

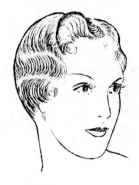

1932

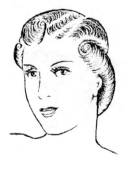

1936

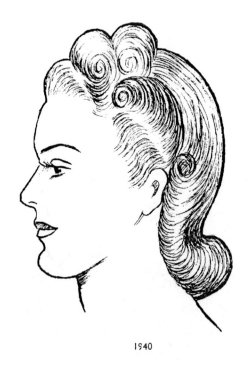

1940

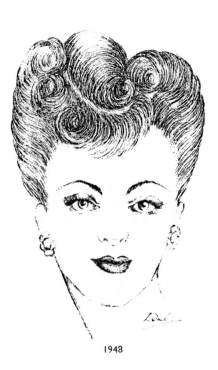

1948

MODERN HAIR FASHIONS INFLUENCED BY HISTORICAL HAIRDRESSING

A final word for that great Frenchman Croisat, who by his personal efforts saved the trade at a time when the Chinese fashion had impoverished hairdressing to such an extent that people looked upon it as ruined.

Croisat sought a method and a fashion with a view to saving the trade and those engaged in it. He studied all historical coiffures; having carried out this laboured study from ancient Greece to ancient Rome, early Christian to the middle ages, Louis XIV, XV, XVI and the First Empire, he found that none of those fashions was to his liking. He then created a style which would please customers and the coiffeur.

When this style was fashioned, the attractiveness and effect were soon admired. Within a few years this 1830 coiffeur became the vogue and brought custom back to the Hairdresser.

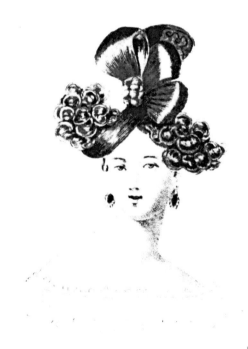 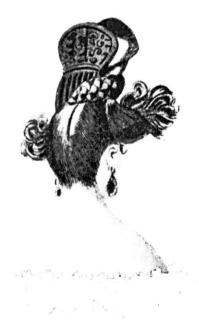

1830

Panorama of Fashion

T HE accompanying illustrations show clearly the evolution of fashions. These fashions form the basis of the artistic side of our profession. As I have mentioned elsewhere in this book, to-day's styles are, for the most part, influenced by yesterday's fashions. Present modes are created by adapting the previous styles to present-day requirements. This applies equally to hair designing and dress designing. fashions which repeat themselves over a period of years.

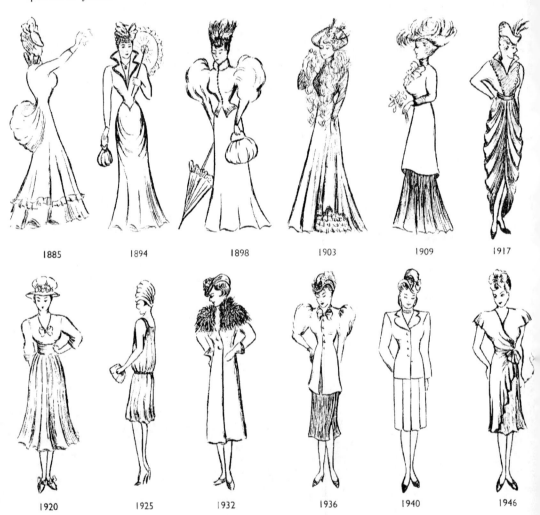

| 1885 | 1894 | 1898 | 1903 | 1909 | 1917 |

| 1920 | 1925 | 1932 | 1936 | 1940 | 1946 |

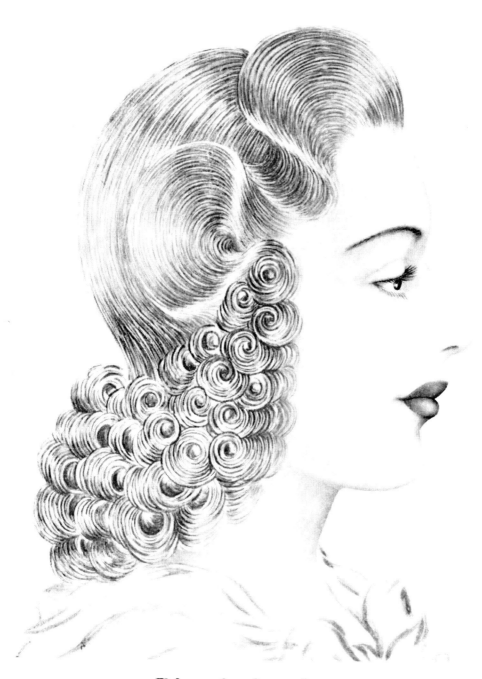

Discrimination

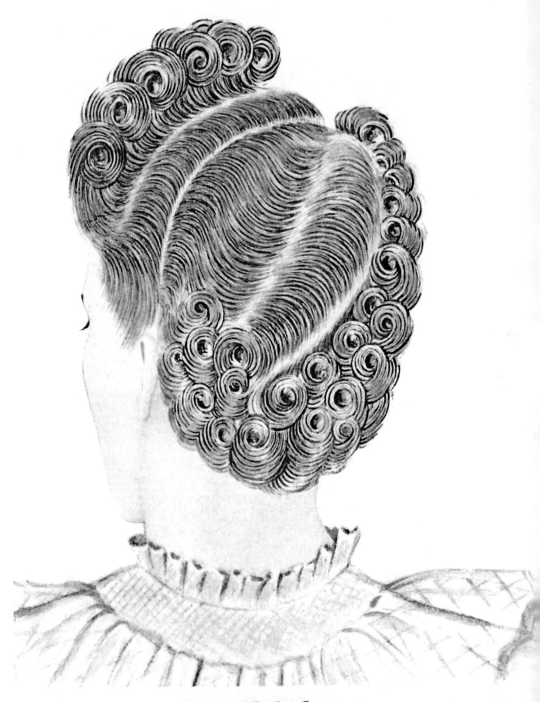

Melody

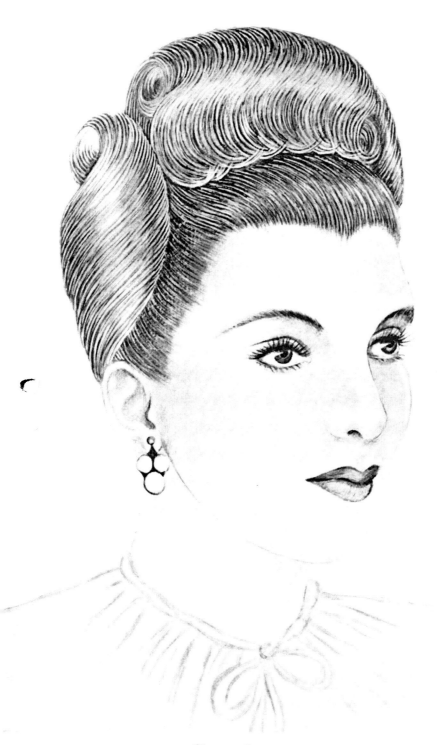

Continentale

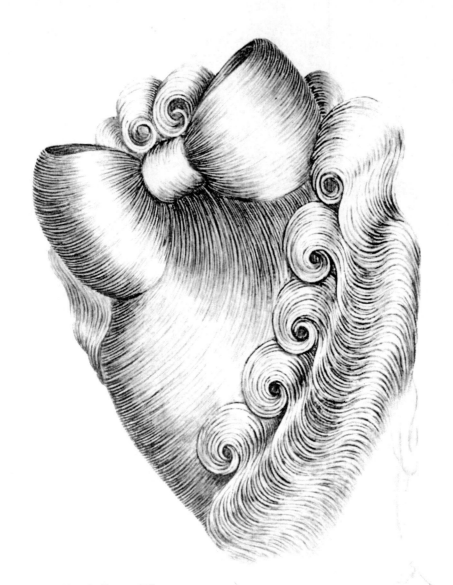

Individuality

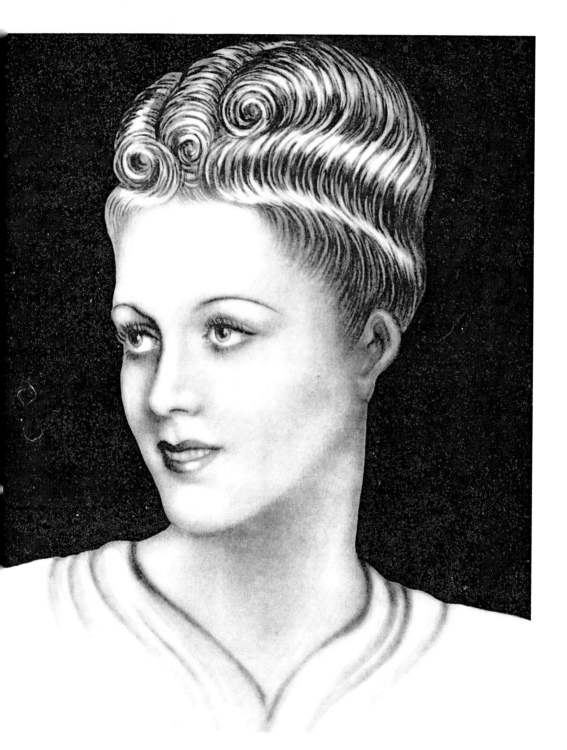

Sumptuous

Vanity Fair

Dear reader, if as far as this you've read,
Consider hair upon a woman's head,
Since Cleopatra—glorious brunette
Entranced Mark Antony with wave and set—
Kings, princes, thieves and poets debonair
Have hymned their praise of a hank of hair
Realms and riches are swayed by glamour
Witness Dubarry, Nell Gwynn and Lamour
So 'tis not strange how patient ladies are
In seeking beauty like a guiding star.
Their face, their fortune, they must all endure
The wildest whim of fashion and coiffure.
For some to give their Love's desire an edge
Are cut and pruned like ornamental hedge.
Some shaped like hearts or fans, some round
Happy their jealous rivals to astound.
And in their mirrors they must always see
Some new extravagance or fantasy
Of upswept waves with breaking crest of
    curls
To break the hearts of baronets and earls.
Some pin their hopes up high with brooch
    of pearl
Others their languid tresses low unfurl.
But all alike in strange and mad pursuit
Since Eve first tasted the forbidden fruit.

Hair Designing Chart

(FOR TRACING)

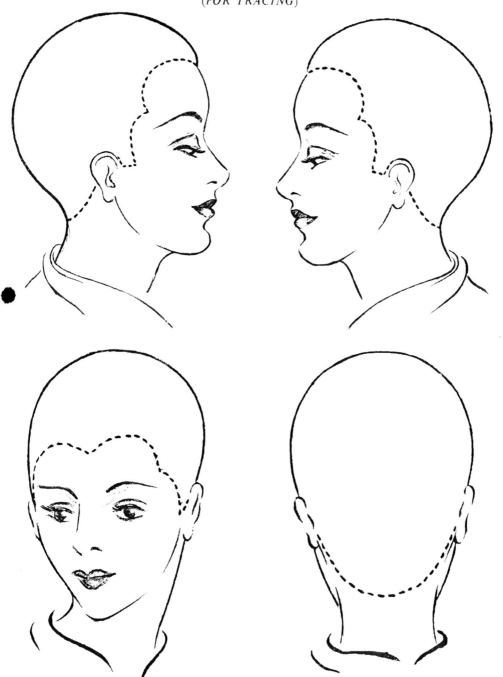

CPSIA information can be obtained
at www.ICGtesting.com
Printed in the USA
FFOW01n0759070116
19976FF